The 16-Word Diet

A Survival Guide for Dieters

By Jay Wiener

For my wife Sharon, my best friend and partner from the time I was 17 years old. I married up.

And for my brother Hap, who succeeded with the most difficult goal of all: he lived a beautiful, complete life.

Acknowledgements:

I have four partners who built a website around my algorithm for ideal weight. and made it possible for hundreds of thousands of people to learn about their ideal weight and lifestyle. More important, each man supported my efforts for years. Thank you to Steve Schlosser, Willie Grief, John Alburger, and our Gatesian Chief Architect Rolland Hoyt.

I would also like to thank my witty and beloved editor, Kate Jones. Visit her at www.gamepuzzles.com, and send her Belgian chocolates.

Contents

Introduction

Don't Start to Diet

The 16-Word diet is more than a book about weight loss; it's a survival guide. So let's begin with a surprise: Don't start to diet. I'm serious.

Start by Choosing Achievable Goals

Most dieters never choose reasonable goals. Worse, they do no planning before they start, unless you count reading the directions on a bottle of magic diet pills as planning. And yet, if those same people wanted to go on vacation, they would prepare carefully. They would choose a destination, book a hotel, purchase plane tickets well in advance, buy some clothes, and then pack their things a day or two before they left. Shouldn't a new lifestyle be planned as carefully as a vacation to Disneyland?

It almost never is, because people almost never understand a basic fact: losing weight is not about food.

It's not about the foods you should eat or the foods you should not eat. It's not about the foods you should only eat after 4 PM or foods you must eat raw or magic foods that will make you strong and virile and young forever or foods that can hook you like heroin or... Enough. Losing weight is not about food. It's about you.

It's about how you live your life every day, forever. Food is an important part of your life but not the only part, and similarly, it is an important part of your weight loss program but not the only part.

And that's why this book is so different from other 'diet' books. It doesn't focus on what you eat; it focusses on how you can live a slimmer, healthier life for the rest of your life, regardless of what you eat.

Three Paragraphs About the Author, and One About You

I'm the mathematician who developed WeightZone, (www.weightzonefactor.com) the scientific alternative to the old Body Mass Index. I've also fought my own battle against obesity; I've stabilized more than 100 pounds below my maximum weight. Better, I did it AFTER I turned fifty, an age at which most people find their bodies in a slow-motion landslide and watch helplessly as their boobs droop down to their belly buttons. I was successful (with both my weight and my boobs), and regardless of how old you are, you can be successful, too.

What does 'successful mean? I didn't simply *lose* weight; I've *stabilized*. That's essential. I had two common motivations: I had my first heart attack while in my forties, so I was driven to be healthier; also, I wanted to look better, after a lifetime of always being the fattest person in the room (or maybe the city). Perhaps most important, I never pretended that I could diet and exercise my way back to the body I had as a muscular teenager growing up in a beach town. That's ridiculous.

About ten years ago, I decided to try one more time – if I failed, I would simply stop trying. I then spent three full months (seriously!) thinking about how to lose weight and how to keep it off. Along the way I established realistic, achievable goals.

You can be successful, too. Are you trying to lose three sizes for that wedding/bar mitzvah/communion/reunion/clothing-optional-booze-cruise that you are going to attend three weeks from Saturday? I can't help you. Do you want to lose weight and maintain it for years, until it becomes your new normal? Keep reading. And while you do, remember that this isn't a diet book; it's a survival guide. And it's fun to read. Not as much fun as a clothing-optional booze cruise, but fun.

Too Much Information

If you are obese and searching for help, you will be bombarded with nutrition information that's partially – or completely – false. You'll be naked in a blizzard of BS, trying to keep your eyes open long enough to spot a butterfly. Diet books lie and diet websites lie and diet programs lie, starting with the promise (wink-wink!) that they have the only solution that can restore the glorious body you had in college.

They will tell you that your problem is too much fat in your diet. Or not enough protein. Or too many carbs. Or not enough healthy fats and oils or too much sugar or not enough fiber or too much wheat or not enough exercise or the wrong types of exercise or not enough water or too much soda or not enough sleep or too much sleep or not enough vitamins or the wrong mix of phytonutrients and certainly the wrong mix of gut bacteria, which means that your own bowels are the problem.

Sure.

Unfortunately, most authors of popular diet programs are willing to merrily transform themselves into quivering piles of gut bacteria in order to sell their books. They use junk science to influence you, not legitimate research, and they devote 100% of their efforts to telling you what you should eat and should not eat, instead of improving your dieting and maintenance skills.

Do you really need to study a scientific explanation about how the insulin mechanism works, or a list of the 250 healthy species of bacteria most commonly found in the human intestinal tract? Worse, do you honestly believe that there is a magic pill containing a magic herb grown in a magic valley that will make your excess pounds disappear while you watch *The Price Is Right*? I hope not, because the full-of-magic-diet-herbs-books and the full-of-unnecessary-diet-technology-books are all full of something else.

One more thing – a pet peeve of mine. The best diet books are astonishingly dull – they can put you into a coma. The best-selling books (rarely the best books) are written as if the readers are junior high students who were left back twice. I think topics this important should be written for adults, and they should be fun to read. I did my best. I hope you'll agree.

A Survival Guide for Dieters

To be successful, you don't need magic and you don't need recipes; you need survival skills. Specifically, you need skills that will teach you how to live a healthy life at a significantly lower weight. For example:

- How do you prepare yourself before you start to diet? (Yes, you must prepare first.)

- How do you choose reasonable, achievable goals?

- What are the most common mistakes people make when starting a diet? (That's three topics and we haven't discussed your ideal food program yet. Get ready:)

- How do you choose between low-fat and high-fat diets?

- What do you need to know about sugar and fat? (No technical jargon or confusing chemical lessons, just practical advice.)

- What makes people slip after months of success?

- What is the true value of exercise to your body? (Seniors – take note.)

- How can you handle weight-loss plateaus?

- How do you stop bingeing?

- How should you manage vacations and holidays?

Ten important topics (there are many others) and only one specifically describes the food plan you should choose. Think of it this way: most diet books are like a new car manual. Colorful and pretty, but useless. The 16-word Diet will teach you how to compete in the Indy 500.

You're at the starting line.

Chapter 1: Prepare to Diet Before You Start to Diet

Okay – I can hear you thinking, "I don't want to prepare – I want to start! Right now!! Where are the 16 Words? What Are They?? When Can I See Them??? *I WANT THEM NOW!!!*"

Slow down, cowboy. Has a hyper-enthusiastic start ever worked for you in the past? Of course not – you gained everything back, every time. In truth, most diets fail before they start. People pick a date to start The Big Diet, but that's all they do. They don't investigate different diet plans, they don't think about an exercise program, and sadly, they don't do anything that's any different from the last Big Diet. And so they fail. Again.

What are they doing wrong? They think they are dieting like Albert Einstein, but in reality they are dieting like an old cartoon character.

Why We Act Like Wile E. Coyote

Recently I watched a **Wile E. Coyote cartoon**. I hadn't seen one in years – decades! – and I loved it. The basic plot never changes: we know how the story begins (craftily), we know how it will end (badly), and every time the coyote falls off a Mount Everest-sized cliff it seems funnier. Except to Wile E.

The poor coyote is obsessed with a dopey-looking bird called the Road Runner. Wile E. doesn't merely want to catch the bird; he wants to conquer it by any means necessary. He plans insanely elaborate ways to trap the Road Runner but they all fail. He builds an infinite variety of WMBDs (Weapons of Massive Bird Destruction) but none ever work; instead, frayed bungee cords snap in his face and enormous rocks fall on his face and bursting dams drown his face and colossal bombs blow up in his face. And every time, the Road Runner sprints away, oblivious to the destruction all around him, merrily chirping "Beep – Beep!"

Hilarious, especially if you are a ten-year-old boy sitting in a dark movie theater – or think you still are.

Like Wile E., we are obsessed with our weight. We want to conquer it. We attempt an infinite variety of Weapons of Massive Fat Destruction, from all-protein diets to all-pasta diets to all-algae diets to worse, but nothing ever works for long. Instead, the diets blow up in our faces while that slender body we are pursuing sprints away, always out of reach.

Why do we fail as often as Wile E. does? Because, like him, we refuse to learn from our past mistakes. We try the same unsuccessful techniques over and over, expecting that this time the result will be better, but it never is. It's the classic definition of insanity and it never will change, unless we change.

If you want to stop falling off those Mount Everest-sized cliffs, start by figuring out which of your behaviors keep failing. For example, if you plan to start dieting on Monday, ask yourself why this Magic Monday will be different from your last ten Magic Monday flops.

Magic Mondays, Magic diet pills, and magic diet books are giant rocks suspended in mid-air, waiting to crush you. If you keep repeating the same mistakes, then you are about to get a massive, Wile E. Coyote-sized headache. This time, do something smarter. Diet like an adult.

Here's a short series of steps that will allow you to take charge of your weight and health forever. After this outline, we'll look at each step closely.

Additional Reading:

Road Runner Cartoon: http://www.wimp.com/a-new-looney-toons-animation/

৶৽৶৽৶৽৶৽

Outline of the Program

Below are short descriptions of the basic concepts of the program. I'll discuss them in detail in the next chapters. Don't skip any, and take them in order. Let's get started.

1. **STOP GAINING WEIGHT.** Don't go on a diet immediately; instead, learn how to stop gaining weight. If you don't, then what will you do when you stop dieting?

2. **START TO EXERCISE.** If you do not exercise, now is the time to start. People who do not exercise look unhealthy and undesirable. What good is a diet if you end up thinner but remain unhealthy and undesirable? Why should you exercise first and diet second? Because you can start walking right now. You'll feel better in just a few days, and walking will become an important part of learning how to not gain weight.

3. **SET REASONABLE GOALS.** Most people have unreasonable expectations about how much they should lose and how quickly they should lose it. If you want to maintain a weight loss, you need reasonable goals for both diet and exercise. Start by learning your WeightZone (www.weightzonefactor.com). Retest yourself every few months, because regular exercise may change your Zone.

4. **SELECT THE DIET THAT IS BEST FOR YOU.** I recommend a protein-centered diet with little sugar, lots of fruits and vegetables, and limited grains, but some people prefer a low-fat diet. Your body, your decision.

5. **LEARN THE 16 WORDS.** Start with the basic rules, then learn how to apply them:

   a. Eat reasonable portions of fresh, healthy foods.

   b. Avoid processed foods and sugars.

   c. Get regular, vigorous exercise.

These are the sixteen most deceptively simple words you may ever read. We will go over them in great detail in Chapter 3.

6. **START TO DIET (AT LAST!)** I understand that this list sounds crazy – you want to start dieting this minute and lose all of your weight by Thursday. However, a diet is like a marathon run. If you do not train for it, you will fail. The first five steps focused on training; now you can start The 16-Word Diet.

7. **LEARN THE ART OF DIETING.** Yes, dieting is an art, difficult to master. The basics are easy: eat these foods, not those. But how do you handle stress? How do you regain control after you have overeaten for a few days or weeks? How do you manage people trying to sabotage your program?

8. **EXERCISE, EXERCISE, EXERCISE.** I discuss exercise throughout this book, and I frequently advise those of you who do not exercise to stop reading and go for a walk. Non-Exercisers: if this advice gets annoying, then you are a S*l*o*w*-*L*e*a*r*n*e*r.

9. **DON'T LOOK FOR MAGIC IN A BOTTLE.** Nothing sold over-the-counter works. It doesn't matter if it's diet supplements, diet pills, diet drinks, diet patches, diet extracts, or a book promising magic food combinations, they are 100% fake. Regardless, there's a steady stream of liars promising that their new product works miracles.

10. **LEARN TO FORGIVE YOURSELF WHEN YOU OVEREAT.** Of all the steps above, this is the hardest. However, this book can help you gain the wisdom to teach it to yourself.

Let's begin by looking at the first step: stop gaining weight. Why? Because you know how to lose weight (you've done it many times) and you know how to regain weight (you've done that just as often). What you don't know is how to do something very difficult: how to stabilize.

So, off to Step 1: how to start. As usual, the first step is always the hardest.

Chapter 2: Your First Day

Start with a Good Plan

I often refer to The 16-Word Diet as 'Dieting for Adults'. That adult behavior starts now. Don't wait until the weekend is over; start now. Not to diet, to prepare. Children rush off thoughtlessly to do something; adults think it through first.

Again, you will not see this advice anywhere else. Most diet books front-load their suggestions so that people lose a great deal of weight very quickly and then, in a premature flush of enthusiasm, convince their friends to buy the same book. However, fast weight loss inevitably fails: it doesn't prepare people to live in a thinner body that is hungry most of the time. And the faster you lose, the hungrier you will be, long-term.

To me, speedy weight loss is a childish appeal to the emotions that has failed all of us before. That's why I advocate an adult approach: prepare yourself to lose weight before you start to diet, so that you can stabilize at a lower weight forever. Start with four goals that you can accomplish immediately. If you want to do them all today, fine. If you want to work on one goal per day, that's fine, too. Your progress is what counts, not the speed of your progress. Your four goals, as described in the last chapter, are:

1. Stop gaining weight
2. Start to exercise
3. Set achievable goals for weight loss and fitness
4. Choose your preferred diet: low fat or low carb

Let's look at each goal in order.

৯৯৯৯৯

Step 1: Stop Gaining Weight

The most common question I get about The 16 Word Diet is, "How can I keep the weight off once I lose it?" The surprising answer is, 'Learn how to stop gaining weight before you try to lose weight." I'm serious.

Stabilize first, lose second, or else you'll be back riding the Weight Loss Roller Coaster.

Stabilize first, lose second. A simple idea, but revolutionary in the stagnant diet industry, which hasn't had a truly new concept in decades. "Learn how to stop gaining weight before you try to lose weight." I repeat that sentence frequently; some people are S*l*o*w – L*e*a*r*n*e*r*s. Not you, of course.

Stop Gaining Weight

Do not diet? It's a startling concept in a video-game-shaped world in which we expect everything to flash-happen instantly, but remember, losing weight is the easy part. We've all done it countless times. Keeping weight off is an extraordinary achievement – about 96% of us fail repeatedly. You need to learn how to do it *before* you get thinner and have to struggle with your new body every day.

The problem is that your body doesn't want you to stay thin. It will fight to regain the pounds you have lost by releasing a flood of chemicals that trick your brain into believing it is starving for sugar.

The result: if you simply go on a diet without proper preparation, it will just be a matter of time before you gain it all back. Again.

Don't wait until you reach your goal; start by taking several weeks – or several months – to learn how to hold your weight steady while you begin to lead a healthier lifestyle. Otherwise, you will fall back into the cycle of losing and gaining, losing and gaining.

A Rarity: A New Idea in Weight Loss

Most likely, you've never heard that advice before. Unfortunately, neither have most experts. Think of all the hyper-energetic weight loss 'experts' you have seen on TV, touting their latest books and promising to teach you a new, magical way to make your extra pounds disappear. Has any expert ever told you not to diet? I didn't think so.

The average diet guru spends his or her time telling you how wonderful his magic diet is or how wonderful he is, but never mentions that he is an unqualified idiot. (Dr. Phil, meet Dr. Oz. Now go away.) That's why popular diets are all temporary fixes for a permanent problem.

The 16-Word Diet

If you follow The 16 Words, you will stop gaining weight. They are all you need to stabilize your weight for life. (I haven't gained any weight for almost 14 years.) The beauty of The 16 Words is that you can use them for diet or for maintenance; the only difference is in how you define "reasonable portions". Start by eating enough fresh, healthy food to stay at your weight today, and then, when you are certain that you can live that lifestyle forever, simply eat a little less. For the first time in your life, you will be properly prepared to diet. Once you learn maintenance, you will develop a wonderful sense of empowerment. You'll be able to eat safely for the rest of your life.

And your life will be better. Occasionally, you'll be able to eat reasonable portions of dangerous foods without triggering a food binge. You won't wake up fearing each day, never knowing if an urge to gorge will suddenly force you into a tiny corner of your mind, hovering above your own body as you eat 10,000 calories in an hour.

You'll be able to socialize without being 'the lovable fat friend who is always on a diet'. (I used to be that guy. I hated it.) You'll be able to take vacations without worrying that after you come home, you will overeat for months. You will have the gift of a normal life.

My Personal Breakthrough

This 'stabilize first, lose second' concept became clear one sunny afternoon more than ten years ago. My son was getting married in three weeks and I had just regained 46 pounds after losing 60. I was wondering what I could do to make those 46 pounds magically disappear, and then reality hit me. Hard. I was wandering in circles, losing and gaining, going nowhere.

Grudgingly, I accepted a sad fact: I would have to wear my fat clothes to my son's wedding. It was September; I decided to not diet again until January 1st. I choose modest goals: to stay where I was, to stop stressing about how to diet, and simply to stop gaining weight. I didn't know it, but I had found a clear path forward after years of being lost.

It was the smartest decision I've ever made. I regained control of my body. Soon after Christmas, I began to lose weight steadily and I've never gained anything back since. Now it's your turn.

The Challenge

Permanent weight loss is very challenging – you'll have to defend yourself against frequent ambushes from your friends, from your family, and toughest of all, from yourself.

You'll be fighting two separate battles, one with your old habits and one with your body. Your old habits probably include eating too much sugar, processed foods, junk foods, fast foods, and not enough fresh, healthy foods. Your body has become dependent on them and they are literally forcing you to stay fat. You're normal.

Many forces Drive Overeating

I can't possibly list all the forces that drive you to overeat – this book isn't long enough. Some have been well-understood for decades, some are new. For example, for decades we have known that overeating sugar will slowly destroy the insulin-producing mechanism that regulates sugar levels in your blood. Low blood sugar can force anyone to overeat massive amounts of sweets.

Other problems with poor eating habits are recently discovered, such as unhealthy digestive bacteria in your intestines. If you eat too much sugar and saturated fat, you will grow colonies of bacteria in your gut that demand a steady supply of both. Seriously. If the little beasties don't get enough, they will manufacture chemicals that ooze into your bloodstream and race to your brain, creating a cascade of painful effects that will not stop until you eat more.

Again, I can't list the many forces that drive you to overeat. Do you want to restrict your calories so drastically that in addition to combating hunger you must fight chemical warfare in your own body? Wouldn't you rather wait and allow your body to naturally heal itself first?

The Simple Solution

Select a healthy style of eating that you can live with forever, not some fad diet that your best friend saw on an Oprah rerun from 1997. Learn how to control your own body by eating fresh, healthy foods while occasionally eating foods you like. Begin to exercise, or start exercising harder. Take your time, follow *The 16-Word Diet*, and don't try to lose weight until you and your body are both ready. Stabilize first, diet second.

Step 2: Start to Exercise

Okay – you are beginning to stabilize. What's next?

- Start to diet? *Wrong.*
- Select the best diet for your body and lifestyle? *Better, but not yet.*
- Ask your friend which diet she thinks is best? *Funny.*
- Go online to find the best new diet pill? *Funnier.*

Seriously – what should you do right now? Start to exercise. It's too soon to diet – you are still learning how to stabilize. While you do that, let's help you feel better (and give you a better body) by exercising.

Stop laughing!

I don't care if you haven't exercised since Ronald Reagan was in office – start now. Today. If you lose weight but do not begin an exercise program, you will go from being fat and undesirable to being thin and undesirable. And the thin part won't last.

Exercise First, Diet Second.

Why? Your goals are to look and feel better, and weight loss is just one of many tools you'll need. If you start to exercise today, then you will feel better today. If you start dieting today, all you will feel is a headache. Dieting will become easier after just a few weeks: exercise helps control blood sugar, which helps control how much you eat and how you feel. Will your hunger disappear? Fat chance. But it will decrease, and your energy levels will increase.

There's another reason to begin to exercise before you begin to diet: serious weight loss requires serious planning; a new exercise program does not. You can start in five minutes: put on good walking shoes and then walk for twenty minutes at a pace that leaves you breathing a bit harder than usual. Do that simple task several days each week and you will be astonished at how it will change you.

Are you too old, too tired, or too busy to exercise? No, you are not. No healthy person is too old or too busy to begin an exercise program. You'll start to feel younger after just a few weeks and your tiredness will vanish – exercise will give you more energy.

Four Easy Ways to Work Exercise into Your Busy Life:

- If you are deskbound, Google "EXERCISE AT YOUR DESK".

- If you walk a lot at work, Google "EXERCISE MY UPPER BODY WHILE WALKING".

- If you are on the road frequently, Google "EXERCISE WHILE TRAVELING FOR BUSINESS".

- If you are busy raising small children, Google "EXERCISES FOR MOMS WITH TODDLERS".

And if you do not work or raise small children but cannot exercise because you are always busy shopping with your friends, going to events, and deciding whether to have two glasses of wine or three with dinner, you don't need to Google anything. You can get all the exercise you need by struggling to pull the top of your body out of your bottom.

The best way to create a custom exercise program is with a certified personal trainer, assuming you can afford one. Just be careful: a good trainer will cost several thousand dollars a year. Trainers are everywhere, but there are far more losers than winners (like E-Harmony). Many trainers have college degrees in a relevant area of fitness; but most have – at best – a high school diploma and they wouldn't know your deltoids from your dad's Delta 88.

Inexpensive exercise classes are available at the local YMCA or Jewish Community Center (both are non-sectarian) and the quality is usually excellent. Also, you can join one of the 'boot camps' that are springing up around the country. Here in the San Francisco Bay Area we have excellent programs, such as the ones run by my friend and colleague Becky Williamson, who is both a trainer and a kinesiologist. Find one close to your home by Googling "BOOT CAMP (YOUR CITY)". Australian readers can visit pages such as http://www.bootcampsaustralia.com/

Later in this book there is an entire section devoted to exercise, but I wanted to get this message out early. If you do not already exercise on a regular basis, stop reading and go for a walk. I'm serious – nothing in this book is as important for your long-term health as is moving your body. You will see this message several times – it is very important. When you come back from your walk, we'll talk about how to set smart goals for yourself.

ھ۰ھ۰ھ۰ھ۰ھ

Step 3: Set Reasonable, Achievable Goals

Next on today's agenda: set reasonable, achievable goals for your weight loss and exercise. Why? Because you cannot diet successfully if you don't have a smart end-point.

Most people pick impossible goals for weight loss and exercise – I see it every day. Middle-aged women want to weigh what they weighed on Prom Night, even though they have three kids. Men try to strength train at the same weight they lifted in college, even though they graduated twenty years ago and haven't lifted anything heavier than a corn dog since then. And of course, just about everyone tries to lose more weight than they should, faster than they should, by eating less than they should. I call that 'Dieting Like a Horny Junior High School Student'. You're already learning a better way: Diet Like an Adult.

Select a Realistic Goal Weight (and Ignore both the BMI and the Waist Ratios)
Start by picking a reasonable goal: the high end of your WeightZone

(www.weightzonefactor.com). (Note: if you are unfamiliar with WeightZone, you can learn about it in the appendix at the end of this book.) Briefly, WeightZone is a mathematical algorithm I researched and wrote; it uses 25 facts about you (body stats, health history, exercise history) to determine your healthy *range* of weight. It will be very valuable as you work your program. I suggest that you learn your Zone as soon as you can.

Obviously, it's better to get the opinion of a professional than to accept numbers from a website, but be careful: most 'professionals' know almost nothing about weight loss. If your doctor mentions your BMI or uses a weight chart, fire her. I'm serious. The Body Mass Index is voodoo medicine, and any doctor or trainer who uses it should lose his license. The ratios that involve your waist measurement are only slightly better; like the BMI, they are useful for describing the health of large groups of people, not individuals.

Think of it this way. Many heavy smokers have smaller waistlines than the rest of us. However, they often die young, after a painfully slow decline. Did their slender waistline help them? Any doctor or trainer who uses waist measurements to provide serious medical advice is poorly informed. Find someone smarter.

How Quickly Should You Lose Weight?

In my experience, the faster most people lose weight, the faster they will gain it back. Quick weight loss is fine for people who gained weight recently, such as pregnant women, vacationers, etc., but if you have been obese for decades, don't expect to lose all of your weight in a few weeks. Your best choice: diet for a while, lose about 5-15 pounds (2-7kg), stabilize at your new weight, and after a few weeks, start again. Repeat that pattern until you are at a healthy weight.

Stabilization is key. Every time you teach your body to maintain a new, lower weight, it will become your new maximum weight. You will never weigh more than that again. Are you unhappy about taking so long to lose weight? Tell me – did losing weight rapidly ever work for you before? Of course not. Dieting is like sex. Slower is better.

Your Goal: Stress-Free Weight Maintenance

Eventually, you will stabilize at a healthy weight and your body will tell you, "You're done." This might be a little above the high end of your WeightZone or it might be lower; don't worry about it.

Note: WeightZone will help you with your exercise goals, too. It analyzes your data and then creates a customized workout schedule based on your health and present exercise patterns. As you read through this book, you will learn how to begin working out after decades of inactivity, and how to make exercise a part of your life. Start slowly, and as your endurance grows stronger increase the speed and intensity at which you work out. Exercise is like sex. Faster is better.

Step 4: Select The Diet That's Best for You

Learning to choose the best diet for your body isn't hard, yet most people are still searching, like Ponce De Leon, for The Enchanted Fountain of Skinny.

The Internet offers countless books and sites, all pushing minor variations of a low-carb diet and most selling enchanted fountains of something: enchanted liquids, enchanted shakes, enchanted pills, or enchanted ideas, such as "You should never eat fruit after 2 PM." (No, I don't know how they handle Daylight Savings Time, but I'm sure the solution is magical.)

The truth is that there are no magic diets, no magic programs, no magic solutions. Despite acres of hype, there are only three types of diets: Low-Carb, Low-Fat, and Low-Calorie. Every diet book on the market is a variation of one of these three. People who choose low-carb (protein centered) diets have a slightly better long-term success rate, both with their weight and with their health, but the choice is yours. Take your time, experiment with all three if you like, and then choose the one that you can live with forever. Not for a few weeks, not for a few months, FOREVER. Why? Because if you ever go back to the way you are eating today, you will regain everything you have lost.

Don't worry – you don't need to know anything complicated about proteins, fats, or carbohydrates; you just need to know which foods are rich in them and which aren't. For example:

Carbs: Sugar is pure carb; fruit juice is almost pure sugar, save them for your birthday. Whole grains such as wheat, corn, oats, and rice are mainly carbohydrates, but they don't affect your blood sugar as badly as sugar does. Fruits have a bad reputation, but they release their sugar slowly, and have little effect on blood sugar.

Protein: Tuna canned in water is almost pure protein. Fish, poultry, eggs, cottage cheese, and tofu are other excellent sources. On the other hand, steak gets its calories mainly from... fat. A juicy sirloin is two-thirds fat and one-third protein.

Fat: Fats are not evil, despite what your skinny-best-friend-who-smokes-too-much says. Vegetable oils and the oil in fish are generally considered heart-healthy and important on any diet. Olive oil and avocados have especially healthy fats. Fats from meat and poultry are in a gray, murky area – new studies keep providing confusing information. However, processed meats put the 'foo' in junk foods.

Eat them only on national holidays, like the Holy Day After Election Day, when they all shut up. Here's a list of healthy low-fat foods.

Dieters have no Enchanted Fountains of Skinny; in fact, we have no Enchanted Fountains of anything. We're stuck with basic science and common sense. Below is a simple description of the three basic diets, to help you choose the best diet for you.

Is A Low-Calorie Diet Best for You?

Let's start with some confusing facts. Low-cal is both the best and the worst way to diet. Historically, it is the most common and the least successful way to diet. And every diet is – ultimately – a low-calorie diet.

Low-cal dieting has a simple philosophy. Eat whatever you like, as long as you eat less calories than you burn up. In theory, you can have your favorite foods and lose weight, too. The problem is that this approach almost never works. Do you know anyone who has ever lost a significant amount of weight and kept if off by simply cutting back on calories without carefully choosing what they eat? Just about no one ever has, unless you want to count the Donner Party.

Why is the track record so bad? People on low-cal diets generally start with healthy, carefully planned meals, but gradually shift to small portions of foods they like. They eat too much sugar and refined flour, not enough fat, and they don't reserve enough calories for good nutrition, which means they feel hungry all the time. You can live with hunger for a week, maybe a month, but not for a lifetime.

Most low-cal diets do not control blood sugar properly, a second powerful reasons that people feel hungry so often. And the low-cal diets that you find online almost never adjust for the caloric requirements of the individual dieter, so big people and active people are seriously deprived of both calories AND nutrition.

There are no links in this section, which isn't an oversight. **I do not recommend any of the classic low-calorie diets.**

Is A Low-Fat Diet Best for You?

Low-fat diets appeal to people who are happiest with a diet that emphasizes fruits, vegetables, grains, legumes, and salads while reducing or eliminating fatty meats, cheese, oil-based salad dressings, cooking oil, nuts, avocados, etc. It can be a wonderful, healthy way to live. However, there are two big dangers. Many people on low-fat diets find that they are hungry all the time, and others have trouble managing their blood sugar. (Some diabetics do very well on low-fat diets; others fail miserably.) Worse, most low-fat diets turn into high-sugar diets. It's almost unavoidable.

Dr. Nathan Pritikin was the first author to popularize the low-fat lifestyle and Dr. Dean Ornish is perhaps its best-known advocate today. Ornish takes a holistic approach to weight loss. He says that you need to change your entire approach to wellness instead of simply going on a diet. That is excellent advice, and his program of diet, exercise, and meditation is very sound – if you have the money, time, and education to support it. However, if, say, you are a single mother working to put herself through nursing school while grandma babysits, then Ornish's program will always be out of reach.

My main argument with Ornish is that he is convinced a low-fat diet is the only path to good health, and refuses to accept that protein-centered programs are effective and healthy. To me, that is unscientific dogmatism. If you are obese, any eating plan that (A) gives you good nutrition, (B) insists that you exercise, and (C) allows you to maintain a healthy, stable weight indefinitely is superior to the way most people live today. You need a healthy eating plan that works for you – not for your doctor.

Is A Low-Carb Diet Best for You?

A Low-Carb Diet (often called The Atkins Diet or a Protein-Centered Diet) is simply a diet in which meat or another protein is the center of almost every meal. Fat is reduced but not eliminated; sugars and grains are minimized. Many studies have shown that this diet is the best choice for most people; its success rate is highest by a small but significant margin. Long-term, it is excellent for controlling both diabetes and heart disease, and most important, it won't leave you feeling hungry all the time. However, it can become monotonous if you reduce carbs too strictly. Strict high-protein diets have a huge failure rate.

Protein-centered diets were controversial for decades, and Dr. Robert Atkins – the most famous advocate – was publicly mocked by most leading authorities, including the once-respected, now-irrelevant doctors Dean Ornish and Nathan Pritikin. The American medical establishment strongly backed low-fat diets, worried that if people ate too much saturated fat, it could lead to heart disease, stroke, cancer, and worse. (What's worse? Dunno.) However, the Establishment was wrong. All low-fat diets led to was a general recognition of the nutritional incompetence of the American medical establishment.

For at least ten years, the news about protein-centered diets has been consistently positive. Study after study has shown that a protein-centered, reduced-carbohydrate diet can lower blood sugar dramatically and improve cholesterol levels and other markers for cardiac events.

For Protein-Centered Dieters, the Basic Rules for Eating Carbs Are:

- Have small portions of any carb.

- Avoid sugar in all forms, including honey, maple syrup, and additives.

- Limit your total intake of grains (wheat, rice, and corn) to one or two ounces a day, max. Less is better, especially if you are a small person.

- Understand that you will occasionally break the above three rules.

Yes, diet rules were made to be broken. Do you honestly believe that one day you will flip a magic switch and then never have another chocolate bar for the rest of your life? I don't. But I do expect to never have chocolate more than once or twice a month for the rest of my life, and I haven't for more than ten years.

On a low-carb diet, you can have reasonable portions of beans, lentils, potatoes, or fruit, if protein is the centerpiece. Can you have two of them? Sure. Can you have all four in addition to a chicken-fried steak? Absolutely. Let me know how it works out.

If your weight boomerangs up and down, and if you keep sticking with one of the three basic diets above, it's time to re-evaluate. Try changing your diet – it isn't working! Also, if part of your boomeranging has included slingshotting from diet book to diet book, then remember that every diet book written during the last forty years has been an inconsequential variation of the same low-carb message, often paired with frequent pitches to purchase some magic crap that the author is trying to peddle.

Remember that diet books are all the same – they take your money but they never help you find The Enchanted Fountain of Skinny. Stick with The 16 Words.

ৡৡৡৡৡ

The 10 Worst Ways to Start a Diet

Before we look at The 16-Word Diet in detail, let's look at some of the mistakes we have all made. Why? So that you never need to make them again. Also, they are a lot more fun than reading about Robert Atkins and Dean Ornish.

1. **Select an Unreachable Goal.** Few things are more pathetic (and more hilarious) than seeing someone trying to lose an impossibly large amount of weight in an impossibly small amount of time. Rapid weight loss is a technique used by high school cheerleaders, jockeys, and people getting ready to go on Tinder. It never works. Do you want to lose weight before some major event? Three points: First, you won't lose nearly as much as you want to lose. Second, you will gain it all back as soon as the event is over. Third, no one at the event is going to look at you unless you are either the bride or a stripper.

    Think about this: how many times have you tried to lose weight quickly and failed? If you want to go on yet another crash diet, then you are a S*l*o*w*-*L*e*a*r*n*e*r. This time, try to l*o*s*e*-*w*e*i*g*h*t*-*s*l*o*w*l*y. If you do, it will not c*o*m*e*-*b*a*c*k*-*q*u*i*c*k*l*y. Got that? Good job!

2. **Believe in Magic Monday.** At some point during your last food-fest, you thought, "I'll start to diet on Monday." How do I know? Been there, thought that. Before you start your next Big Monday Diet, ask yourself a few questions: Why is this Big Monday Diet going to be any different from every other Big Monday Diet? What planning have you done to make it different? What have you learned to make it more successful? And what is a 'Big Monday Diet'?

3. **Try to lose weight before you learn to maintain your weight.** What is the point of dieting if you don't know how to keep the weight off? Sooner or later, you'll need to stop losing weight and remain stable for the rest of your life, which is nearly impossible. You cannot learn how after you lose weight, while your body is desperately trying to sabotage you into regaining those pounds, so you must learn how to stabilize before you start to diet. Again, I'll discuss this in detail later – it is an essential part of The 16-Word Diet Program.

4. **Start to diet without a plan.** This one is hard, but it is the heart of this list. Some people start to diet with less thought than they give to deciding which summer rerun to watch on TV. They

rarely make it past Magic Monday. Does this sound as if I am repeating myself? You are not S*l*o*w.

5. **Don't Exercise.** Diet miracles won't happen while you sit and watch TV. I have a friend who used to complain that he looked like a bloated bag of crap. One day he went on an all-liquid diet and stuck with it for months, but he never got around to exercising. Pretty soon he looked like a wrinkled bag of crap. And then he gained all his weight back. Now, he looks like (let's say this together) a bloated, wrinkled bag of crap. He does this periodically, because he is a S*l*o*w*–*L*e*a*r*n*e*r.

    Another, more serious note: obese people who eat healthy foods and exercise regularly tend to live longer than 'normal' weighted people who do not exercise or eat properly. If you do not exercise, then please stop reading this and go for a walk. I'm serious.

6. **Take Diet Advice of Any Sort from Your Best Friend.** I say this with love: your best friend is an idiot. Note: My dear friend and editor Kate J. suggested that the word 'idiot' is too strong. She doesn't know you as well as I do. So please supply your own descriptive noun: Don't take diet advice from your best friend because your best friend is an _*_*_*_*_. Good job!

7. **Buy low-fat processed foods.** Memorize this easy factoid: low-fat processed foods are made by removing fat and adding sugar. If, at this point in the book, you do not know that sugar, not fat, is what makes us gain weight and develop heart disease and diabetes, then you really are a s*l*o*w*-*l*e*a*r*n*e*r. Read the ingredients list on food that you want to buy and then ask yourself, "Would I give that stuff to my dog?" If the answer is 'yes', ask yourself, "Why do I hate my dog?"

8. **Smoke marijuana to 'relax'.** Few things are less relaxing than the frenzied orgy of unstoppable eating that starts after you smoke a joint. That's why I stopped smoking grass in the Eighties. I miss marijuana almost as much as I miss bell bottoms.

9. **Don't eat enough fruits and vegetables.** People have been telling you to eat fruits and vegetables since Mom started to feed you mushy baby food. If you still haven't listened, then you are a s*l*o*w*-*l*e*a*r*n*e*r. First, fruits and veggies are loaded with essential micronutrients (you know that). Second, the fiber in fruits and vegetables is essential – among other things, it slows down and reduces food absorption, so that your body takes in fewer calories, with no insulin rush. Third, the sugar in fruit will not affect your diet. Finally, if you are still drinking fruit juice and smoothies twenty years after every responsible nutrition expert told you to eat whole fruit and use your juicer as a doorstop, then you are the s*l*o*w*e*s*t*-*l*e*a*r*n*e*r I know.

10. **Take Diet Pills You Bought Online.** Over-the-counter diet pills do not work. It doesn't matter if they are sold online or in a store, it doesn't matter how many carefully coached celebrities endorse them, diet pills do not work. Ignore the amazing success stories and the before and after pictures – they are fictional stories about fictional people. More absorbing than *50 Shades of Grey*, but less realistic, which is hard. Easy question: do you know anyone who lost weight and kept it off by using diet pills they bought over the counter? I didn't think so. So why waste your money trying to find Magic in a Jar?

11. **Cut too many calories.** If you cut too many calories, your body goes into starvation mode. You will be sleepy, move slowly, and stop burning many calories. The weight you lose will be mainly water (which will come back in a few days), and muscle tissue (which may be the dumbest thing to do on this entire list). What you will not lose is fat.

12. **Give up after you cheat.** Human beings make mistakes. All of us do. If cheating sends you into a frenzy of guilt, please print out these words and paste them on your refrigerator: **Sooner or later I am going to cheat on my diet. And then I'll stop cheating and start dieting again.**

Okay – the above is what you shouldn't do. (Believe me, there's more coming.) Now, let's get serious.

Chapter 3: The 16-Word Diet

You have accomplished a lot after reading just two chapters:

- You learned the value of planning your diet before you start to diet.

- You began to teach yourself how to stop gaining weight – a major accomplishment.

- If you already exercise, you've improved your program.

- If you didn't exercise, you started a modest program. Congratulations – that is the most difficult achievement in this entire book.*

- You have selected reasonable, achievable goals for weight loss and exercise.

*If you have not yet started to exercise, what the hell are you waiting for? Get off your butt and go for a walk. *Right now.* I don't care if you are reading this on a plane full of screaming babies and garlic-eating adults – get up and walk around until the stewardess whines that you are in the way.

That felt good.

ৡৡৡৡৡ

The 16-Word Diet – The Basics

Now that you understand the differences between a Low-Fat Diet and a Low-Carb Diet, I'll explain why the differences aren't very important. What matters most are The 16 Words. Seriously.

Years ago, when low-carb was making yet another comeback, I began to wonder why some people succeed with low-fat diets while others do better with low-carb. The best foods on one are the worst on the other, yet people succeed with both. How could this be?

My surprising conclusion was that, done correctly, the two diets are almost identical. The problem is that almost no one does them correctly.

Most people understand that on a low-fat diet, the most important rule is to avoid fat. Butter, cheese, fatty meats, etc. Pretty simple. And wrong. Similarly, most people understand that on a low-carb diet, the most important rule is to avoid carbohydrates: fruits, grains, and sugars. Wrong again. Think about it this way: if those guidelines were all that are necessary, most people would succeed. However, most dieters have lost weight with both regimens and then gained it all back. The low-something guidelines failed them. And yet, a few ordinary folks, indistinguishable from the crowd, have been successful.

Why? It helps to start with a brief history.

If you are under forty, you may not know that low-fat diets are a relatively recent fad. During the Fifties and Sixties, low-carb was the rage. Some books sold millions of copies: The Drinking Man's Diet, The Scarsdale Diet, The Doctor's Quick Weight Loss Diet, and in 1970, the megahit **Dr. Atkins' Diet Revolution** made 'Atkins' a household name. (Note: I was a patient of Robert Atkins, we became friendly, and I consider him a mentor.)

However, during the 1950s, a persuasive scientist named Ancel Benjamin Keys began promoting the concept that diets rich in fat caused obesity and heart disease. He was astonishingly successful despite having little data to back up his theories. He ran studies that would be unacceptable today, but no one challenged him; few doctors are qualified to evaluate statistical techniques. By 1980, the entire medical establishment was promoting low-fat eating to prevent or even cure most major illnesses: heart disease, diabetes, even cancer.

People began to look at fat as if it were poison. Serving fatty dishes to friends became almost as socially unacceptable as smoking cigars at the dinner table. However, if the host served a sugary fruit compote for dessert, she would be applauded for avoiding fat. And overnight, the country got fatter than ever.

Around 2000, low-carb diets swung back into fashion. Well-designed studies documented that protein-centered eating was as healthy as low-fat and had a higher success rate. Dr. Atkins, a medical pariah for decades, was recognized as a pioneer.

There was only one problem: as the country lurched back towards low-fat dieting, the obesity epidemic continued to grow.

And so today, we have chaos. Utter confusion. A few people succeed with low-carb diets, a few with low-fat. Medical doctors promote low-fat diets while medical researchers promote low-carb. And nothing seems to help the vast majority of dieters.

What is going on? Simple: It isn't a specific food plan that allows some dieters to succeed; it is everything else they do.

Why Are a Few People Successful?

What do these people do that helps them keep their weight off for years? Simple. They don't avoid a few specific foods; they avoid an unhealthy life.

Consider the basic instructions for a low-fat diet: avoid fats, avoid processed foods, and get regular exercise. Now, consider the basic instructions for a low-carb diet: avoid sugars, avoid processed foods, and get regular exercise. There is a one-word difference. If we weren't living in a food-obsessed society, the similarities would be obvious.

This is wonderful news. You can stop your fruitless search for the 'perfect diet' because the eating plan that works best for you is perfect – for you. Also, you won't need to waste your money every time you find a new diet book written by some poor clown trying to turn himself into a rich clown; the diet books are all the same. (Except for this one, of course. You should buy copies for all of your friends. I desperately want to be a rich clown.)

The specific diet plan does not matter – both low-carb and low-fat work. Low-carb has a slightly higher success rate, long – term, but that might not be true for you. Choose the one you find easiest to stay with, permanently. What matters is what you eat and how much exercise you get. If you get plenty of exercise and eat modest portions of mainly healthy, unprocessed foods, you will lose weight and stay healthy. Not glamorous, but it works. Doubt me? Try to find a healthy junk food addict who maintains a significant weight loss, or a healthy couch potato who keeps her weight off and has a terrific figure. You cannot do it.

People who exercise regularly and eat healthy foods will always be healthier than their sluggish, sugar-slurping friends. That includes many people who weigh a bit more than society would like: those extra pounds turn out to be protective. 'Slightly overweight' people live longer, with fewer health problems, than do thinner or heavier people. (FYI, that last sentence describes me perfectly, although I'm stretching the word 'slightly'.)

Additional Reading:
Can We Say What Diet Is Best for Health?

ॐ~ॐ~ॐ~ॐ~ॐ

16 Words, 3 Rules

So... if there isn't a major difference between low-fat and low-carb dieting, how should you proceed? The preposterous claim in the title of this book is true: everything you need to know about losing weight permanently can be explained in sixteen words. Three rules, sixteen words.

1. **Eat reasonable portions of fresh, healthy foods.**

2. **Avoid processed foods and sugars.**

3. **Get regular, vigorous exercise.**

These sixteen words completely describe every successful, long-term weight loss. The specific food plan is immaterial; what counts are the three rational rules. The 16 Words work.

Perhaps the best part is that you can start today. Right now. You can actually follow them while you decide if you do better with low-carb or low-fat. *You can (and should!) follow them while you learn to stabilize – they will make it much easier.*

Either way, the 16 Words will keep you successful forever. I watch my carbs (low-fat diets kept me hungry all the time), but you should choose whatever works best for you. Just remember that you are eating for your body, not anyone else's, so your opinion is the one that counts.

Spend the coming weeks deciding which fresh, healthy foods to eat, long–term. While you do, reduce your dependence on processed foods to an occasional desperate treat, even if that means that you must (argh) cook for yourself. It's worth it. And if you do not exercise, start today. Go for a walk right now, then finish this when you come back. (Note: I plan to keep saying that until you listen.)

That is the essence of The 16-Word Diet. Nothing flashy, no miracle solution that no one in the entire world knows except for me, just common sense. As you read this book you'll learn how to lose weight and improve life from the inside, without fad diets, preposterous rules, worthless pills and supplements, or worse.

৬৯-৬৯-৬৯-৬৯

Breaking Down The 16-Word Diet

Let's look at the 16 words again:

1. Eat reasonable portions of fresh, healthy foods.
2. Avoid processed foods and sugars.
3. Get regular, vigorous exercise.

These three rules contain six separate ideas:

1. Eat reasonable portions

2. Eat fresh foods

3. Eat healthy foods

4. Avoid processed foods

5. Avoid sugars

6. Get regular, vigorous exercise

Let's look at each idea in depth.

Eat Reasonable Portions (Portion Control)

Portion control is the toughest part of dieting. Let's make it easier.

Everyone knows a woman who wants a trim body like Giada De Laurentiis but who has an appetite like Joey Chestnut. And everyone knows a man with Joey's appetite who wants to attract a woman like Giada. That's why portion control is so difficult: we are rarely rational about the amounts of food we eat, especially while we are dieting.

When I started writing about diet and exercise, no one asked about portion control. Most questions were variations on the same theme: Which diet is better – low-carb or low-fat? The unexpected yet obvious answer (the best diet for you is the one you can stick with for life) led me to write this book. And that's when the portion control questions started.

What is a Reasonable Portion?

The problem was with Rule #1: Eat reasonable portions of fresh, healthy foods. People kept asking, "What is a reasonable portion?" Frankly, I've never known how to define one. I studied what the experts suggested and came to an unexpected conclusion: the experts didn't have an answer, either.

Nutrition experts suggest two different ways to determine correct serving sizes: use a scale to measure food by weight, or use a portion control device that lets you measure by eye. The problem is that the standard guidelines for weight are useless and the portion control devices were designed for guppies.

I dismissed the portion control devices immediately. They only come in one size, but people come in many sizes. A scale made more sense, and I thought the US Department of Agriculture websites would help. Big mistake: the USDA is located in Washington, DC, but it dispenses advice from 1972. The USDA – controlled by Big Agriculture and staffed by earnest little people who live in Munchkin Land – still recommends elfin portions of a low-fat diet based on grains. And white bread is fine.

I clicked away, even though I miss 1972.

Diet Professionals Give Amateur Advice

The National Institutes of Health have a friendly explanation of portion sizes, but only if you are less than 14 years old or if your IQ is under 80. For the rest of us, the explanations are... uncomfortable. Next, I searched the Mayo Clinic website as it promised to demonstrate what a serving of protein looks like. It proudly shows a small, dry piece of broiled chicken breast, the type of protein portion that prison wardens give to dwarfs doing hard time.

I kept looking.

Everydayhealth has a page called Ten Easy Portion Control Tips. Paydirt! They suggest hummingbird-portions of everything, but they offered clear, easy-to-follow ways to estimate serving sizes. A one-ounce serving of cheese is the size of a domino. A one-cup portion of vegetables should be the size of a tennis ball. This was great! Except... I own a tennis ball. And I own a measuring cup.

I dropped the tennis ball into the measuring cup; it wasn't close. I Googled the volumes of each: the ball holds about 8 cubic inches (131 cc) but the cup holds about 15 (246 cc). I could probably squeeze two tennis balls into a cup if I shaved off the fuzz, and the pile of fuzz would make a perfect Mayo Clinic serving of something.

The cheese/domino comparison was worse. Was the writer referring to tournament-sized dominoes or the ones we buy at Toys-R-Us? The tournament size is much larger than the home size. I did some field research. In my refrigerator. After reducing most of a two-pound brick of cheese down to shrapnel, I ended up with a perfect, domino-shaped, one-ounce portion. It was almost twice as big as my grandchildren's dominoes, but much smaller than the tournament pieces. Apparently, the Everydayhealth.com writer flunked fourth grade math.

Dieting for Adults

But I noticed something interesting. Somehow, my little block of cheese looked as if it weighed one ounce (28 gm.) It wasn't a reasonable portion (unless you are tiny and sedentary), but I instinctively knew it weighed an ounce. My wife said the same thing, while helping to clean up the shrapnel. She said it was just common sense. And then I understood: the best way to determine portion size is with common sense. All the advice about weighing food and measuring food is Dieting for Dummies. If you are a regular reader, then you prefer Dieting for Adults.

Instead of worrying about a perfect calorie count, just relax. Then, when you fill your plate, use common sense.

- First, remember Rules 1 and 2 of *The 16-Word Diet*: Eat fresh, healthy foods, and avoid sugar and processed foods.
- Second, drink a glass of ice water just before you eat. That will make it easier to keep your portions small.
- Third, before you start to eat, look at your plate for thirty seconds.

Thirty seconds is a long time – long enough to calm down and take control of yourself before you eat too much. It's also long enough to decide how much of the food on your plate you will eat. My grandfather fought obesity fifty years ago and his rule of thumb still applies: eat half of whatever is on your plate, wait a few minutes, and if you are still hungry, eat half of whatever is left. And as soon as you are no longer hungry, STOP EATING! That is what I do (most of the time) and it works.

If you do purchase a portion control system, please write to let me know about your progress. I don't think you'll end up looking like Giada De Laurentiis, but if you do, send me a picture.

****

On a very different note, Joey Chestnut, mentioned in the first paragraph, is a professional competitive eater. (Yes, there is such a thing.) In July 2016, he ate 70 hot dogs in ten minutes to win a national hot dog eating championship at Nathan's in Coney Island. I bust a gut to write 40 free posts a year and Joey didn't bust a gut while stuffing down 70 hot dogs. And he won $10,000. And he has groupies. I hate Joey Chestnut.

Now that we've had some fun, a final thought. The suggestions above may not always be enough to reduce your portion sizes with any consistency. Fortunately, a few of the recent generation of portion control devices may actually work for you. My favorite is the one designed by my friend Amanda Clark. I discuss it in detail here:
http://www.weightzonefactor.com/blog/how-portion-control-helped-me-

lose-weight-without-dieting/. Her system is simple but effective, her advice and recipes are professional and hype-free, and I use it myself – it has helped me lose 15 pounds or so during the last year. However, other good products are available, and my goal is to help you lose weight, not to sell something. Here's a link to an **Amazon** page that offers a few alternatives to Amanda's system: http://amzn.to/2f8pJG1.

ఞఞఞఞఞ

Eat Fresh Foods

Here in California, the fresh food movement began shortly after **Balboa** discovered the Pacific Ocean. Today, we casually shop in supermarkets offering a variety of meats and produce that would have astonished our grandmothers.

I have close friends who moved here from Moscow in 1990, during the collapse of the Soviet Union. They found it very difficult to adjust to the vast array of food available everywhere. In the USSR, people waited in line for hours to purchase items as mundane as bananas and mangos. In Russia they were exorbitantly priced and rarely available; here unlimited quantities are available every day, for pocket change. Fresh foods are a gift. Take advantage of it.

How Do You Define 'Fresh"?

First and most important: the fewer steps between the farm and you, the better. If food came directly from the farm or the ocean, it is fresh and healthy (usually). If it was frozen but otherwise unprocessed, it is almost as healthy. Meat, fruit, vegetables, and dairy are all in this category. Saturated fat will not be an issue if you follow the 16 Words.

At the other extreme are prepared meals in the frozen foods section. Pick up a box of frozen corn dogs and read the ingredients list. After you get past the usual fats, sugars, and chemical sludge, you may see the words 'chicken shit' in very small letters. And even if you don't, remember that inspiring additive the next time you want to microwave, say, a box of hot wings and French fries and call it dinner. Do you really want to put all that chicken shit into your body?

Grains are healthy, too, if you eat them whole – before they are processed in some fashion. Steel cut oats are fine; quick-cooking oats are not. They are the oat-equivalent of white bread: instant oatmeal may raise your blood sugar and make you hungry.

Is bread healthy? Be careful. Bread is highly processed. The whole grain bread you bought so virtuously this morning comes from grains that were dried, ground into flour, stored in an unrefrigerated warehouse for days or months, blended with a variety of sugars and preservatives, baked, stuffed into a bag while still warm enough to absorb a distinct *fragrance plastique* and finally, after sitting on a supermarket shelf and being squeezed by a dozen shoppers before you, it ended up in your shopping cart. Still want that toast?

Here's my suggestion: don't eat too much bread, and have 100% whole grain most of the time. Eating white bread occasionally is fine, as long as you eat other grains, too. And fresh produce, obviously.

How to Shop in The Supermarket

I'm just guessing here, but you probably don't think you need guidelines about how to shop in the supermarket. However, if a recovering alcoholic had to go to a liquor store to buy wine for a New Year's Eve party, wouldn't he establish guidelines for himself first? Why are you different? I'm serious. This is a book full of flippant remarks, but not this time. If you have had a long-term weight problem, how are you different from that recovering alcoholic? I'm not. Alcoholics and addicts are my brothers and sisters, even though I've never been addicted to any drug harder than chocolate fudge.

The simple trick to buying fresh foods, from the great Michael Pollan, is to purchase food from the displays on the periphery of the store – the walls – and to avoid the aisles. The walls are where you will find fruits and vegetables, meats, poultry, and fish, the dairy section, and high-end breads. (Yes, you're going to purchase bread so you might as well get the best. Again, buy mainly whole grain breads and eat it sparingly.) The periphery is the place to be adventurous – and to save money. Often, fruits and vegetables go on sale when they are at their peak of ripeness – when they are healthiest and most abundant. Some things are dicey; for example, farmed shrimp from Asia should be banned from the entire country, but they are an exception. In general, the periphery is the section of the supermarket that will keep you healthy and thinner.

Supermarket Interiors Are Not Your Friend

The frozen foods aisles are chock-a-block full of delicious, unhealthy foods – the most delicious, least healthy assortment of foods ever available in history. Even The Donner Party had a healthier diet, although I don't recommend it. Frozen food cases are generally in the center of the supermarket, which isn't an accident; that's where the highest profits are. Enter your favorite store and walk straight towards the back, soon you will be surrounded by frozen desserts and frozen pizza and frozen Chow Mein and frozen-delicious-everything. Few things taste better than processed frozen foods – I know; I've tried them all. That's why for years, my wife and I have avoided the frozen foods section whenever possible. Our trick? We don't browse. We plan ahead and only buy the items on our list - mainly frozen vegetables, which are fine, although not as tasty as fresh. We never buy frozen juice, which is one of the least healthy products in the store.

Okay – the periphery is healthy and the frozen foods are dangerous. What about the other aisles?

The other aisles are mostly stocked with crap: canned crap and bottled crap and powdered crap and ethnic crap and instant crap and sugary crap and sugar-free crap and mountains of toilet paper. For all that crap.

There's very little on these aisles that you need more than occasionally. Canned beans, rice and other grains, peanut butter, and a few other staples, that's all. Stick to your list and you will be fine.

One last thing. Just because something is fresh doesn't make it healthy. If you eat honey a few hours after a bee keeper harvested it, it is fresh, delicious sugar that can be toxic in large doses. Worse, filtered honey can come from any source, usually China, despite the label, which means it could be adulterated with anything. Fresh sushi is delicious but dangerous; raw fish can give you a variety of intestinal parasites and worse. Fresh produce should be properly washed before you eat it; it could be contaminated with a variety of unspeakable bugs from a variety of unspeakable sources.

You get the picture.

ৡৡৡৡৡ

Eat Healthy Foods

How can you tell if a food is healthy? Easy. If you aren't sure, it probably isn't. The more something is processed, or the more unpronounceable ingredients you see listed on the label, the more likely it is that you are looking at dog food in a pretty package.

Often, the initial reaction to "Eat reasonable portions of fresh, healthy foods", is "If food is fresh, it must be healthy, right?" Not exactly. Whipped cream is fresh and unhealthy, beans are dried and healthy, so use your judgment. Especially if you are eating beans.

If you aren't sure, what should you do? The answer is in the first three words: "Eat reasonable portions". Think about butter and margarine. Starting in the 1950s or even earlier, we were told, "Butter is unhealthy. Eat margarine instead." Then, fifteen or twenty years ago, we were told that margarine is made with trans fats, which are very unhealthy, and ten years ago researchers began to find that butter isn't so bad for us after all. It's both confusing and funny. However, if you stick to a single pat of butter, little harm can be done. In fact, if you stick to reasonable portions, almost anything fresh is healthy. Just stay vigilant about what and how much you are eating, and you'll be fine.

ھ۔ھ۔ھ۔ھ۔ھ

Avoid Processed Foods

"Dried beans aren't fresh. Are they processed?" No. The rule is, "the fewer steps between the farm and you, the better." Dried beans are harvested, washed, dried, and packaged. That's pretty straightforward. No fats or salt are added, no stabilizers, preservatives, gums, flavor enhancers, food dyes, etc. By contrast, think about processed chicken. A piece of chicken – white or dark – is very healthy. However, a piece of ground chicken that rode an assembly line on which it was coated with thick breading, fried in a vat of old oil, and then doused in "orange flavored sauce" is suitable for maggots, not you. Don't let it near your body.

Check out the nutritional label from Tyson Chicken Nuggets:

Nutrition Facts: Serving Size: 5 PIECES (90g) Servings Per

Container: About 4

<u>*Amount Per Serving*</u>

Calories from Fat 160 Calories 270

<u>*% Daily Values**</u>

26% Total Fat 17g, 20%, Saturated Fat 4g, Trans Fat 0g, Polyunsaturated Fat 6g, Monounsaturated Fat 6g, 13%, Cholesterol 40mg, 20%, Sodium 470mg, 5%, Total Carbohydrate 15g, 0%, Dietary Fiber 0g, Sugars 0g, 28%, Protein 14g

Ingredients: Chicken, water, wheat flour, contains 2% or less of the following: brown sugar, corn starch, dried garlic, dried onion, dried yeast, extractives of paprika, natural flavor, salt, spices, wheat starch, white whole wheat flour, yellow corn flour. Breading set in vegetable oil.

There are 270 calories per serving, and 160 come from fat. Just 56 calories come from protein. Now, look at the ingredients. Where does all that fat come from? Not from the chicken – wash off the breading and you'll need reading glasses to see those 4 grams of meat. But at the end of the laundry list of ingredients, it innocently says, "Breading set in vegetable oil." The word 'set' is a euphemism for 'soaked.' Yum. And how about that 'chicken'? Is it breast meat? <u>Pink slime</u>? Tyson isn't saying, so I'm not eating.

Note: just before publishing the first edition of this book, I tested all the links in the online version, including one on the Tyson site. It is gone. Tyson took down all the nutritional informational from its site and replaced it with… Nothing. Looks as if Pink Slime is a good way to describe Tyson Management.

Read the Label

Here are some easy rules for an ingredients lists:

1. If it is a frozen prepared dinner, be very careful. Some are excellent, but most are dog food.
2. If there are a lot of ingredients that you do not recognize, don't eat it.

3. If there are a lot of chemicals that you cannot pronounce, don't eat it.
4. If it gets most of its calories from fat, do not eat it.
5. If there is wording that isn't crystal clear, such as "Breading set in vegetable oil", do not eat it. (What does 'set' mean? I have no idea.)
6. If it is a granola bar, it is probably a candy bar with a little toasted oatmeal stirred in to make you feel virtuous. Do not eat it.

ॐॐॐॐॐ

Avoid Sugars

Avoiding sugars (yes, it is plural) may be the most difficult two words of The 16-Word Diet. Sugar is everywhere and it often hides in unexpected places (bread, popcorn, ketchup, etc.).

Sugar is everywhere and yet it is poisonous. Are you fond of fat-free foods? Friendly, tasty, fat-free processed foods are actually scoops of sugar wrapped in chemical-crud blankets. We all know this and yet, if you were out to dinner with friends and someone said, "Come back to my house! I have a fabulous, fancy, fat-free dessert!", you'd think, "What a great idea!"

No one expects the fabulous, fancy, fat-free dessert to be a bowl of cut fruit. Instead, everyone looks forward to fat-free frozen yogurt or fat-free banana cream pie or fat-free chocolate mousse or something even less healthy, if that is possible. And then everyone feels virtuous about themselves after gobbling down a fat-free, nutrition-free plate of sugar, preservatives, artificial colors, and artificial flavors, blended with a smorgasbord of confounding chemicals.

Processed, Fat-Free Desserts Are Bad for Your Diet

It's clear that processed, fat-free desserts break Rule Two of The 16-Word Diet™, but something deeper is going on. For more than fifty years, we were taught that fat is evil and sugars are harmless. The two concepts were taught as axiomatic truths, despite the inconvenient fact that they weren't. **Both Claims Were Based on Deeply Flawed Studies**. The statistics and the conclusions were inaccurate, but for decades, scientists and researchers who questioned the conventional wisdom were mocked. Living a fat-free lifestyle was drummed into us like a primitive religion.

Today, despite mountainous evidence that the low-fat lifestyle has made the world fatter, all that indoctrination has created an established truth, impossible to leave behind. Our culture has been brainwashed by the fat-is-evil cult; as a result, sugar consumption and diabetes have soared.

Think about this:

- Pure, refined cocaine is extracted from harmless coca leaves. Our ancestors chewed the leaves, fresh and whole, for centuries.
- Pure, refined sugar is extracted from harmless plants. Our ancestors chewed the plants, fresh and whole, for centuries.
- Refined cocaine and refined sugar are both white powders that can kill us. And yet only one is illegal.

What's the danger from processed sugar? Simple. It causes your pancreas to work too hard producing insulin; eventually, it will wear out. If you eat, say, a sugar beet, the sugar will be slowly released over the course of a few hours, as the beet is digested. Your insulin levels will stay low and flat. However, if you drink the same amount of sugar in, say, a glass of Coca Cola, the sugar will hit your bloodstream all at once. Your pancreas will go into overdrive; your insulin levels will soar and then plunge. Catastrophe. Do it once and you may be hungry an hour later. Do it for months and you may gain weight. Do it for years and you may get diabetes and heart disease, so those 50 pounds you gained from eating all that sugar will be just one of your problems.

Sugar Hides Under Assumed Names

Processed food is easy to recognize – just look at the ingredients list. The longer the list, the less frequently you should eat it. However, recognizing sugars is complex. Sometimes it is easy: cane sugar, honey, fructose, high fructose corn syrup, maple syrup, etc. Six different names for poison. But what about Concord grape juice concentrate? Sounds delicious, but it is a fancy name for sugar. Fruit juice concentrates are essentially sugar with a small amount of aromatics added for taste.

And how about anhydrous dextrose, panela, mycose, mylose,

nigerotriose, and nipa sap? All sugar. Literally hundreds of different types of sugars are added to our foods, and you cannot know them all. Here is one hint: if a food ingredient ends in 'ose', it is probably sugar. If it doesn't, it may be sugar anyway. A Facebook page lists <u>329 names for sugar</u>, and the list keeps growing.

Sugar is everywhere. For example, soda is flavored sugar water. And so is fruit juice of any sort; most of the nutrients have been removed. Most breakfast cereals are boxes of sugar and refined carbohydrates with a few nutrients tossed back in to impress mom. There are exceptions, of course: steel cut oats are terrific; however, they take longer to cook. The simple rule for hot cereal: the longer it takes to cook, the better. Instant hot cereal is effectively a bowl of sugar.

Sugar is also a surprising ingredient in many foods, from ketchup to pepperoni pizza. You don't need to avoid these types of foods completely, just watch for them and factor them into your diet.

And that's about it. Sugar and fat-free foods are everywhere and they are bad for you. But you knew that already. You learned the truth about sugar and fat-free processed foods years ago; you didn't need me. So here's my question: if you knew this already, and if I understand it so well that I just wrote about it while watching the Giants beat the Mets in the bottom of the ninth, why do we still eat so much of the stuff? And why will we say 'yes' the next time someone invites us over for a fabulous, fancy, fat-free dessert?

Note: Sugar is too broad a topic for a single chapter. I discuss the dangers of fructose (HFCS) in a separate chapter.

Get Regular, Vigorous Exercise

This is the most important of the three rules of The 16-Word Diet, and yet it is the most neglected. Exercise is the single most effective way to stay healthy and live a long life. That's why, in several places, I make a surprising and sometimes impolite request: stop reading this book and go for a walk. If you don't start now, you may never start. This book can teach you how to diet and exercise, but you have to do it yourself.

Why is exercise so important? Here's an easy question: would you rather be overweight and live a long, healthy life, or be thin and live a shorter, unhealthy life?

The answer is obvious yet everyone gets it wrong. We loudly shout **HEALTHY!** but we secretly want THIN! That's why we all focus on the wrong number: the number of pounds we weigh today, not the number of minutes we exercised this week. Yet exercise, much more than body fat, determines how long we will live, how good we will feel, and how healthy we will be for our entire lives.

Too many people believe that the third rule of The 16-Word Diet applies to other people, not them. How sad.

The third rule is simple and direct: **Get regular, vigorous exercise.** It doesn't say, "Get regular, vigorous exercise or go shopping" or "You can skip this rule." The four words are simple and clear.

Any exercise is better than no exercise, but intensity makes it better. Intense, strenuous exercise improves our bodies in ways that casual exercise will not. Think of it this way. Watching TV with your dog is bad for your body. Strolling with your dog is good. Running with your dog is great. And if you can run while carrying your Labrador, you don't need to read the rest of this article.

Studies Show the Value of Exercise

Two recent studies have shown the importance of stressing your body during exercise. In November 2014, Dr. Paul T. Williams published the results of his monumental National Walkers' Health Study. The study monitored the health of nearly 40,000 recreational walkers for more than nine years, and the results were crystal clear: the faster people walked, the lower their long-term risk of mortality and dementia. When compared with faster walkers, the people who merely strolled (defined as taking more than 23 minutes to walk a mile or 1.6KM) had a 44% increased risk for mortality from all causes and an astonishing five-fold increase in risk for dementia. This was true even if they walked long enough each week to satisfy standard exercise recommendations. The good news: the faster people walked, the lower their rates of mortality and dementia.

It's the best incentive for exercising imaginable.

A second group of researchers published the results of a study that examined the difference between muscles subjected to regular, vigorous exercise and muscles exercised lightly over the same period. As GRETCHEN REYNOLDS wrote, "Intense exercise changes the body and muscles at a molecular level in ways that milder physical activity doesn't match. Though the study was conducted in mice, the findings add to growing scientific evidence that to realize the greatest benefits from workouts, we probably need to push ourselves."

Muscles react differently to intense exercise than they do to light exercise. More important, over time your muscles will grow larger and stronger, and your body will become more efficient at releasing stored fat for use as fuel. Moderate exercise will not do this efficiently.

It's valuable information. The studies also show that you should not get into a rut. Mix up your exercises; don't perform the same routine every day. Why? Because no matter how hard your routine is, your body will eventually learn how to perform it in the least stressful way possible – and your vigorous workouts will become less valuable.

"The point is to get out of your body's comfort zone," said Dr. Michael Conkright, one of the authors of the study, "because it does look like there are unique consequences when you do."

Now for the important part: what should you do? The most important thing to do is this: do not feel guilty if your workouts are not perfect.

Some basic info:

What is Cardio Exercise?

'Cardio' is anything that gets your heart rate up and keeps it up. It's a bit like Viagra, except that if you can keep cardio exercise (or anything else) up for four hours, then you should have written this book, not me. Walking, jogging, biking, swimming, rowing machines, etc., are great ways to get your pulse elevated. Also, tennis, soccer, and basketball provide wonderful aerobic exercise, but baseball is about as stimulating to the heart as watching someone buy a vowel on Wheel of Fortune.

Is Strength Training Important?

Many people walk or run regularly but they do little or nothing for their upper body. Big mistake. First, strength training will build muscles for anyone, even 75-year old grandmas who think they don't need muscles (they need flexibility). Muscles burn calories 24 hours a day – even while grandma is sleeping – so they will help her (and you) burn fat faster. Also, many people past fifty lose not just strength but flexibility. Reaching up to get something from a high shelf becomes difficult; putting on a shirt or jacket becomes painful. Strength training can prevent this, and it can halt or reverse stiffness if it has already started. Also, if you have arthritis, strength training may be the best way to relieve pain and slow down the progression of your disease.

As I mentioned earlier, later in the book there is a complete chapter about exercise: how it can improve your health and looks and how much it can help you lose weight. There's also a section devoted to myths about exercise. But for now, let's continue to focus on The 16-Word Diet.

Summary

The nice thing about The 16-Word Diet is that it makes sense. Simple, reasonable sense. No complicated instructions, no confusing scientific jargon, no *Superfoods You Must Eat!,* no *Evil Foods You Can Never Eat*, no gimmicks about when you should eat your food or the order in which some bonehead thinks you should eat specific foods, etc., just common sense. Eat reasonable portions of fresh, healthy foods, avoid processed foods and sugars, and get regular, vigorous exercise. If you want to lose a few pounds, cut roughly 500 calories per day – less if you are a small, older woman, more if you are a large, active young man. If you go on vacation, accept in advance that you will eat more processed foods and sugars than usual. And live your life.

****

There's one last topic to cover in this section, even though it isn't formally a part of The 16 Words. None of the above suggestions will work well if you do not have a healthy assortment of bacteria living in your intestinal tract. Fortunately, all of the concepts of The 16 Words have the same effect: they help improve digestion by improving your assortment of bugs.

Don't get squeamish: we all have them, and without them your intestinal tract wouldn't work. An unpleasant thought.

ھھھھھ

Maintain a Healthy Microbiota (After You Learn What It Is)

Are gut bacteria important to your health? Yes. Your gut bacteria may be the most important organ in your body that you know absolutely nothing about. Fortunately, the topic isn't gross. (Usually.)

Gut bacteria – often called the "microbiome" or the "microbiota" – consist of thousands of species of bacteria that live together in our intestines, munching away on whatever we eat, often converting it from indigestible to easily digested and absorbed. Not thousands of bacteria, thousands of *species* of bacteria. There are literally trillions of bacteria in our intestines; they are essential for life, not just digestion. Without them, we would last a few weeks at best.

The microbiome – gut bacteria – is so important to our health that many scientists consider it another organ of the body.

Why Gut Bacteria Are Essential for Health

Chapter 95 of the 4th Edition of Medical Microbiology states:

> "Enzymes produced by intestinal bacteria are important in the metabolism of several vitamins. The intestinal microflora synthesizes vitamin K, which is a necessary cofactor in the production of prothrombin and other blood clotting factors. Treatment with antibiotics, particularly in individuals eating a diet low in vitamin K, can result in low plasma prothrombin levels and a tendency to bleed. Intestinal bacteria also synthesize biotin, vitamin B_{12}, folic acid, and thiamine.

> The intestinal flora is capable of fermenting indigestible carbohydrates (dietary fiber) to short-chain fatty acids such as acetate, propionate, and butyrate. The major source of such fermentable carbohydrate in the human colon is plant cell wall polysaccharides such as pectins, cellulose, and hemicellulose. The acids produced from these fiber substrates by bacteria can be an important energy source for the host."

The microbiome is essential for life. Not important – essential. Consider this: the appendix, long thought to be a useless vestigial organ, is now believed to have an essential role in keeping us alive: it evolved to harbor a healthy reservoir of gut bacteria. It stores and nurtures them, so that it can repopulate the intestines after someone survives a disease like cholera that causes explosive diarrhea. (Hey! I can't always write about puppies and sunshine!)

On the topic of things explosive, the research community is blowing up with studies showing that the microbiome impacts almost every area of life, not just obesity.

Heart disease, diabetes, obesity, cancer, depression, mood swings, and other seemingly unrelated conditions are closely linked with the microbiome. It can literally control our actions, even down to choosing the foods we eat.

Sound impossible? Consider this: if you like to feast on, say, sugary donuts, pastries, and cookies, you will build vast colonies of bacteria that like to feast on the worst ingredient in those foods: sugar. Go on a protein-centered diet that eliminates your favorite goodies and the tiny, sugar-craving beasts will begin to weaken and die within hours. As they do, they'll produce chemicals that affect your brain. In addition to developing a colossal headache, you'll feel tired and depressed, and the urge to eat sugary doughnuts and more will be overwhelming.

This isn't the only reason that dieting is so hard, but it's a major factor.

The good news: if you stay on that protein-centered diet (or another sound eating plan) for just a few weeks, you will reduce your colonies of sugar and white flour-loving bugs to insignificance. You'll also encourage the growth of healthy strains of bacteria that specialize in breaking down hard-to-digest foods like fiber.

Yes, you can permanently improve the mix of bacteria in your gut by simply adopting a healthy diet with lots of fiber. And no, you don't need to swear off your favorite donuts, pastries, or cookies forever; you simply can't have them often enough to regrow large colonies of those undesirable beasties.

This explains why it is so difficult to start dieting again after overeating on a long holiday weekend. All that vacation sugar has encouraged the growth of the worst bacteria and suppressed the healthiest. The solution? Get back on a healthy eating plan (not a crash diet!) and stay on it until your gut is back in balance.

Which Foods Encourage Healthy Gut Bacteria to Grow?

To improve your mix of gut bacteria, do four things: Eat reasonable quantities of fresh healthy foods, avoid processed foods and sugars, get regular, vigorous exercise, and eat more fiber. (Maybe I should have called this book *The 19-Word Diet.*)

If you stop eating junk foods, eat mainly healthy foods, and regularly have foods that contain probiotics or prebiotics, you'll starve the unhealthy colonies of bacteria that chomp away on excess sugar and make room for healthy colonies to grow. If you begin to eat fiber, you will feed the healthy bugs, and their colonies will crowd out the unhealthy ones.

Just one thing: you can't get enough fiber by having lettuce on your hamburger for lunch and Metamucil at night. Life isn't that easy. Enjoy fruits and/or vegetables with most meals, and over the course of the month have a wide variety of both – washed but unpeeled. And don't worry about the microscopic residue from fertilizers and pesticides that might be left on the peel; that's neurotic. Worry about global warming, which has begun to drown Florida.

How many veggies should you eat? My friend Cindy Gershen, co-author of The Fat Chance Cookbook, has a simple formula. Cover half of your plate with vegetables, and use the other half for protein and (maybe) complex carbohydrates, or 'starch': potatoes, corn, rice, etc. This should describe not just your dinner plate, but your lunch, too. If that makes lunch at KFC a little awkward, too bad.

How much fruit should you eat? 2 – 4 pieces a day. If possible, keep trying new varieties. Don't worry about the carbs unless you use a juicer; fruit is perfectly safe on a low-carb diet but fruit juice is NOT safe for any diet, ever. An excellent rule of thumb is to average one piece of fruit for every 50 pounds or 25kg that you weigh.

The above three paragraphs are generic; they don't exactly apply to either low-fat and low-carb programs. However, both are easy to adapt: low-fat lovers should minimize the fats used, and low-carb people should minimize the potatoes, grains, etc. Either way, you need lots of fiber – fiber that is added to food isn't very useful, but fibrous plants really do improve your health. Short term, you'll feel fuller. Long-term, you'll feel better.

New Studies Are Being Published Every Day

And now to do something a little unusual: I'm going to shut up. Almost. Research projects and published studies about gut bacteria are important, but there is no way to keep up with them all. I certainly can't write about them all. Instead, here are links to recent studies of the different effects the microbiome has on our bodies. Some might be important to you, some not. You can decide which ones to read.

****

Additional Reading, with short comments:

Artificial Sweeteners May Change Our Gut Bacteria in Dangerous Ways

Last year, a team of Israeli scientists put together a strong case. The researchers concluded from studies of mice that ingesting artificial sweeteners might lead to – of all things – obesity and related ailments such as diabetes. This study was not the first to note this link in animals, but it was the first to find evidence of a plausible cause: the sweeteners appear to change the population of intestinal bacteria that direct metabolism, the conversion of food to energy or stored fuel. And this result suggests the connection might also exist in humans.

Can the Bacteria in Your Gut Explain Your Mood?
The rich array of microbiota in our intestines can tell us more than you might think.

Gut Microbiomes Change During Weight-Loss Surgery, Leading to Benefits That Last a Decade

Losing weight is difficult. Ask a fitness expert and they'll say exercise more. Ask a nutritionist and they'll say eat healthier and curb your portions. Ask a doctor and he might prescribe you a weight-loss surgery. They're becoming more and more popular within the U.S., and new research shows that altered gut bacteria have important link to weight-loss surgery success stories.

Bespoke diets based on gut microbes could help beat disease and obesity

Early trial showed use of computer algorithm to produce diet tailored to a person's unique biological make-up had benefits for pre-diabetic subjects

How Your Gut Bacteria May Influence Your Heart Health

Bacteria living in a person's gastrointestinal tract can influence the health of their heart by affecting their weight, blood lipids and cholesterol levels, a new study reports.

Fecal Transplants Made (Somewhat) More Palatable

Two studies showed that encapsulated pills containing healthy human feces in frozen and freeze-dried form were effective in treating recurrent C. difficile. But it was not clear how to produce the capsules in large quantities.

Your Gut Bacteria May Be Controlling Your Appetite

The microbes in your stomach seem to hijack a hormone system that signals the brain to stop eating.

U.S. Navy Recruits Gut Microbes to Fight Obesity and Disease

The military is creating "smart" E. coli to combat a variety of disorders...

Why drinking red wine and eating chocolate may be good for your gut

Diversity is good for your gut – and red wine might help. In a recent study, researchers from Belgium and the Netherlands present the most comprehensive work on the human microbiome to date. After studying the poop of thousands of citizen volunteers, they've mapped out the species of bacteria that live inside their guts – and linked some of those bacteria to associated lifestyle factors.

Some scientists hope to use the microbes that live in our guts to diagnose and treat the diseases that seem to be linked to them.

Breast milk could give babies bacterial boost

Breast milk could be doing more than just nourishing a newborn – it could also be helping them develop healthy bacteria to protect them from disease, illness and obesity. New research from the University of Colorado Anschutz Medical Campus looked at the role of human milk hormones in the development of a baby's microbiome – their bacterial ecosystem – in their digestive system.

Published in the *American Journal of Clinical Nutrition*, it's the first study to suggest breast milk could shape an infant's microbiome.

40 Trillion Bacteria on and in Us? Fewer Than We Thought.

There are a lot of bacteria on us and in us – our microbiome, it is called. Calculating exactly how many microbes each of us carries is hard, and the most common number cited, both in popular and scientific literature, is almost certainly wrong.

Study of Hunter-Gatherers' Guts Reveals Ancient Microbes

Bacteria found in far-flung indigenous groups are absent in industrialized populations.

After traveling upriver in the Peruvian Amazon, researchers from the University of Oklahoma and Peru's National Health Institute returned with evidence that – when it comes to the bacteria living in your gut, at least – you are what you eat, not where you live.

Can the Bacteria in Your Gut Explain Your Mood?

The digestive tube of a monkey, like that of all vertebrates, contains vast quantities of what biologists call gut bacteria. The important genetic material of these trillions of microbes, as well as others living elsewhere in and on the body, is collectively known as the microbiome. Taken together, these bacteria can weigh as much as six pounds, and they make up a sort of organ whose functions have only begun to reveal themselves to science.

****

The 16-Word Diet is a rare diet book – simple, rational, and gimmick-free. Let's end this chapter by looking at a few examples of… more common books in this genre: faux diet books that were written to make money for the authors and publishers, not to help improve the health of the general public.

❧❧❧❧❧

The 10 Worst Diets of the Decade

A remarkable number of diet books, written by unqualified people and based on preposterous, unscientific theories, have made their authors rich. Why? Because Americans keep gaining pounds but not IQ points. Diet advice has morphed from insanely strict high-protein diets to insanely strict low-fat diets to quickly-lose-tonnage-in-days diets to the latest fad: quickly-lose-weight-and-inches-from-specific-parts-of-your-body diets. The fact that spot reducing is scientifically impossible doesn't seem to matter.

For about twenty years, every new book has offered a minor variation of the 100-year-old, high-protein diet popularly called 'Atkins'. To pump up sales, authors have learned to disguise Atkins by adding a few modern improvements (eat fruit!) or by inventing preposterous restrictions on what you can eat based on the time of day, the season in which you were born, your blood type, or whether you're an innie or an outie.

If you are ever tempted by some new version of Magic in a Bottle; you'll need to be prepared with facts. Remember these short reviews:

1. <u>Burn the Fat, Feed the Muscle</u>: A high-protein diet that targets forty-year old men who think they can look like 20-year-old body builders. Good luck, children.

2. <u>The Raw Food Diet:</u> The perfect diet for people who think that self-flagellation isn't painful enough. People on the Raw Food Diet don't cook anything, including meat. Raw vegetables make perfect sense, but... raw eggs? Raw fish? Raw chicken? These dieters may lose a lot of weight, but so what? Who wants to kiss them?

3. <u>The Glycemic Index Diet:</u> Surprised to see this respectable diet on a list of losers? Alas, it belongs here. The Glycemic Index is junk science. (Typing that sentence broke my heart – I was once a believer.) The GI was a brilliant idea: researchers attempted to rank different foods on a scale of 1 to 100, based on their effect on blood sugar. Unfortunately, the testing procedure was poorly designed, so the results were useless. The <u>Glycemic Load</u> is much better but it remains imperfect; the science is evolving.

4. <u>Shred: The Revolutionary Diet: 6 weeks 4 inches 2 sizes</u> by Ian K. Smith
    Does this mean that if my tiny grandmother and my son the former football player both go on the Shred diet, they will each lose 4 inches and 2 sizes in six weeks?

5. <u>SuperShred: The Big Results Diet: 4 Weeks, 20 Pounds</u>: SuperDitto.

6. <u>The Daniel Plan: 40 Days to a Healthier Life</u> by Pastor Rick Warren. Forgive me for observing the obvious: Warren is a sincere, charming, utterly unqualified weight-loss 'expert' who gets most of his exercise from thumping on a bible.

7. <u>6 Ways to Lose Belly Fat Without Exercise</u> What I like most about this book is the utter shamelessness of the title. It suggests that the author has created an enchanted mix of foods that somehow forces your body to burn fat from the pad over your abdominal muscles before it burns fat from anyplace else. Who throws money at this crap?

8. <u>The 21-Day Tummy Diet</u>: A high-protein diet with specific instructions for people who can't stop farting. You can't make this stuff up! And it might actually work! Just don't write and tell me about it.

9. <u>6 Weeks to OMG!</u> By Venice Fulton
This book actually advertises that "Broccoli carbs can be worse than soda carbs", which may be the single stupidest statement ever uttered by someone who was not an anchor on cable news.

10. <u>The 8-hour Diet</u> ZincZenko and Moore
"Stunning new research shows readers can lose remarkable amounts of weight eating as much as they want of any food they want – as long as they eat within a set 8-hour time period." Wow! This is even stupider than that quote about broccoli carbs. Why 8 hours? Because 9 hours takes too long. Come to think of it, so has this.

Note how many of these books offer massive weight loss in an impossibly short time. Most people don't want to learn how to lose weight permanently; they want magic solutions that require no effort and no pain. The good news: if you have read this much of The 16-Word Diet, you are smarter than most people.

If you ever weaken, just remember that these diet books were not written by serious people; they are fluff written by fluffers for F*l*u*f*f*y*-*L*e*a*r*n*e*r*s. The books are summer beach reads, throwaways bought in an airport and left unfinished on a plane, forgettables meant to give the reader a few hours of false hopes. They are piñatas, stuffed with colorful but useless advice that should be beaten out of them with sticks.

Chapter 4: Time to Start Your Diet (Finally!)

How many diet books do you own? I own at least twenty. What a waste. I could have spent that money on something I enjoy more, like traffic school.

The problem with most diet books is that the author's main goal is to sell more diet books. Helping you lose weight is secondary. He or she wants to sell as many books as they can, as fast as they can, before the next pop diet book pushes them off the Amazon bestseller list. As a result, diet authors all offer short-term advice: lose it fast and don't blame me if you gain it all back. This means that the author must fill about 200 pages with recipes, corny stories about imaginary people, and a Magic Diet that works for everyone and is somehow different from all the Magic Diets that came before it.

The problem with Magic Diets is that they never work for very long. Never. We aren't caged laboratory rats being fed carefully controlled diets; we are human beings with unique bodies. We shop at the mall or go out with our friends or hike on a beach or binge-watch something on TV. And occasionally, we will slip and eat something that is expressly forbidden by whatever Magic Diet we happen to be following. And then we are lost. That's why carefully controlled diets are rarely successful for more than a few months: pop authors never learn from past failures.

The World's Best Diet Is Also the World's Worst Diet

My favorite example: *US News and World Report*. Every year it publishes a new evaluation of diet plans, and every year its experts rank The DASH Diet as #1. They never learn. When illustrated on an attractive spreadsheet, DASH is perfectly healthy: low-fat, low-sugar, and ultra-low salt. The problem is that the diet flops when followed by actual humans, who prefer food that does not taste like an attractive spreadsheet. I humbly suggest that before *US News and World Report* publishes its next evaluation of diets, its experts try to find someone who has actually followed the DASH Diet for longer than, say, breakfast.

Similarly, the USDA teamed up with the U.S. Department of Health and Human Services to produce their 2015 set of Dietary Guidelines, which they update every five years. The guidelines are a definite improvement over the 2010 Guidelines, in that they allow more saturated fats and less added sugar, but then things start to collapse, as the influence of Big Agriculture takes over.

Instead of warning people to avoid soda like Coke, fruit juice like Mott's, and sweet, creamy coffee drinks from Starbucks, The Dietary Guidelines vaguely suggest that we should "consume less than 10% of calories per day from added sugars." Instead of warning about the dangers of eating too much processed meat, it ambiguously advises that we "consume less than 10% of calories from saturated fats" – guidance that is obsolete. Perhaps worst of all, the dangers of hyper-salted, preservative-laden processed foods are never mentioned.

People who follow The Dietary Guidelines, which are based on low-fat, low-sodium meals, are doomed to failure; the Guidelines promote flavor-free dishes that leave people feeling hungry. A modern low-carb diet – vastly superior to either DASH or The Dietary guidelines – is really a lower-carb diet: refined grains and sugars are still off the table, but fruits and modest portions of whole grains are back on. Reasonable portions of fats and oils are perfectly fine – they are not dangerous, despite what we were told for decades, and they will keep you feeling full.

More important, many studies show that protein-centered dieters remain the healthiest, long-term, despite the fat in their diets. True, Dr. Dean Ornish and his low-fat fan club occasionally leave their remote little retirement village (they live in 1974) and make some grumpy noise, but Ornish is roughly as relevant as an episode of Happy Days. (Note: some people do beautifully on a low-fat, low-added-sugar diet. It is a very healthy lifestyle if you are one of the few who can stick with it permanently.)

Time to Start Losing Weight

My suggested program is next. Stick closely to it to lose weight, and then relax a bit to maintain your weight. You'll find no rigid, easy-to-break rules; instead, I'm offering a simple, gimmick-free program for a long, healthy life.

Earlier, when I wrote "Plan your diet before you start to diet", I wasn't kidding. But think about all you've learned since you started. If you took several weeks or months to learn to stabilize your weight, congratulations. You are now stronger and healthier than you were when you started. If you like, go back and reread whatever isn't 100% clear, because now it's time to lose weight.

৯৯৯৯৯

Jay's Perfect Protein-Centered Diet Plan

Here's the diet that I follow and that many of my readers have adopted. No complicated rules, no foods that you must eat or that you must not eat; just common sense. Do not think for an instant that I am the ultimate authority on any of these topics; question everything. Google any topic you want to learn more about; just avoid the sites trying to sell Magic in a Bottle. Also, be sure to go to reputable sites that provide science-based answers and that do not try to sell you diet pills, supplements, or meal replacements.

1.   Eliminate almost all carbohydrates from your diet for 1 to 3 weeks. No longer – you might snap. Depending on your size, physical condition, and on how much you eat, you'll lose 3-15 pounds. Note: **this step is optional**; it will speed up your early weight loss, but does it matter? When I started, I stuck to a high-protein diet for exactly six days plus one breakfast, and then told my wife I wanted a sandwich for lunch.

2.   Have protein as the center of every meal, including breakfast. For how long? Forever. Lean meat, poultry, fish, eggs, cottage cheese, Greek yogurt, and tofu are all excellent sources of protein. Beans, nuts, and legumes are good, too. However, hot dogs and processed meats are fine on July 4th, not every time someone turns on a barbecue. (Of course, if eating ground pig anuses doesn't bother you, you can break this rule.)

3.   How much protein should you eat? The Zone Diet has an excellent suggestion: select a portion of meat that is about the size of your palm. (Fish tends to have fewer calories than other meats, so you can have a larger portion.) This approach doesn't require a scale, and it automatically adjusts to a person's body size; a construction worker will have a portion twice the size of his maiden aunt's.

4. **Enjoy reasonable amounts of fats.** Fat is not the enemy. Recent studies show it will not give you heart disease; the real villain is sugar. Also, fat will keep you from getting too hungry before your next meal – a very good thing. An ounce or two of peanut butter on apple slices, some olive oil over your salad – learn how much fat you need to stay full for 3-4 hours. Obviously, you should avoid things like deep-fried foods, but feel free to use reasonable portions of healthy cooking oils such as Canola Oil. And given the (unlikely) choice between, say, cheese and SnackWell's, eat the cheese and toss away the low-fat SnackWell's. Dairy fats have been shown to be protective against heart disease; low-fat treats are pure sugar, and sugar is pure poison.

5. **Slowly work in a few** healthy complex carbs when you are ready. Beans, lentils, potatoes, yams, parsnips, and fruit are fine, but hold off on any grains for the first few weeks of your diet. No wheat, corn, rice, barley, rye, buckwheat, quinoa, etc. Why? In my experience, dieters who successfully avoid sugars may compensate by overloading on grains. Try doing without them – you will be surprised at how much better you will feel in just a few days.

6. When you are ready to add grains back in your diet, keep portions small, infrequent, and stick with whole grains. Quick cooking oats or white rice are no better than white bread, but steel cut oats and whole grain rice are fine – after a few weeks. A small serving of quinoa has 28 grams of carbohydrate but just 6 grams of protein.

7. **Eat all the vegetables you like,** raw or cooked. If you do not like vegetables, you never had them cooked properly. Boiled or steamed veggies taste like prison food, but if you grill them they taste spectacular. I often have salad with my breakfast eggs, but rarely bread. Why? When I eat bread with eggs (even whole grain), I get hungry by 11 AM. With salad, I stay full for an hour or two longer even though I'm eating fewer calories.

8. **Eat fresh fruit (not fruit juice).** You can eat 1-3 portions of fruit from the day you start to diet, depending on your size. (If you want a fast, initial weight loss, wait a week or two.) The sugar in

most fruit is absorbed over the course of several hours, as the gastrointestinal tract slowly breaks down the fibrous materials that shield the fructose (fruit sugar). As a result, your blood sugar will not spike. Later, when you want to maintain your weight, you can eat more. One good rule for fruit is to average one piece of fruit daily for every 50 pounds or 25kg that you weigh.

9.   **No sugar.** Avoid sugar, honey, maple syrup, corn syrup, candy, soda, fruit juice, etc. They can raise your blood sugar and make you feel hungry, even if your belly is full. Sell your juicer on Craig's List; juicers grind out delicious drinks that are mainly... sugar. Why? They break down plant fiber and release most of the hidden fructose. Even if you drink the pulp, that freed-up sugar will quickly hit your pancreas, which will respond by spinning out insulin like a juicer with the top off. Remember: sugar makes you hungry; fat keeps you full. (Yes, I write that pretty often. No, I don't plan to stop.)

10.   **No highly processed food, junk food or fast food.** How do you know something is junk food? If it comes pre-wrapped and most of the ingredients on the label are unpronounceable, it is junk food. If it comes in a paper bag and you buy it from a fifty-year-old minimum-wage worker sitting in front of a cash register, it is fast food. FYI, that fifty-year-old minimum-wage worker is the sharpest employee in the store. Still want those fries?

11.   **Drink very little alcohol (and drinking none is better.)** A glass of wine every day is the most you should have. Mormons consume no alcohol at all and they live seven years longer than the rest of us. Yes, I understand that a fair amount of research has shown that a glass of wine a day has heart-healthy properties, but more recent studies have indicated that the earlier studies might be wrong. The jury is still out. Worse, many people cannot stop at one glass of wine per day – and so they lower their life expectancy significantly. Worse still, the shorter life expectancy may not matter to men who drink – heavy consumption of alcohol is a major cause of ED. Which may explain why those non-drinking, healthier-than-the-rest-of-us Mormons have so many children.

12. Can you cheat occasionally? Of course. Eating an occasional treat that's not on some list of approved foods isn't 'cheating'; it's being human. Just be sure that the occasional treat doesn't become a nightly event. And finally:

13. Calories count. Not as much as we used to believe, but a lot. If you stick to fresh, healthy foods and get regular exercise but still eat too much, you won't lose a pound. I've done that and you have, too. Also, not every calorie is equal, despite the ignorant old maxim that 'a calorie is a calorie'. Your body will not react the same way to 100 calories from table sugar as it does to 100 calories from lettuce, even though in both cases the calories come from carbohydrates.

Pretty simple. Logical, too. I have followed these rules for years and they keep me at a weight I can live with – a little chubby by choice, but healthy and young. I don't want to spend a lifetime without chocolate or cookies, but I restrict myself to only having them when they are offered to me and never buying them. Your job is to figure out what works for you. If you follow The 16-Word Diet, stick with the program, and be patient, you will never worry about your weight again.

Download printable versions

Two versions of this diet are available online in PDF format. You can download either and print it out:

This version is identical to the diet above.

This is an abbreviated one-page version that you can put on your refrigerator.

Additional Reading:

The following books give excellent guides to a reduced-carb diet you can live with. Just remember not to stay on an ultra-low carb diet for more than a few weeks – that weight loss technique has a 100% failure rate. Note: I purposely chose two old books and just one new one; most new diet books are too gimmicky.

- **The South Beach Diet** Dr. Arthur Agatston

- **Dr. Atkins' New Diet Revolution** Dr. Robert Atkins

- **Fat Chance (2014)** Dr. Robert Lustig

Here are links to studies about the effectiveness and safety of low-carb, protein-centered diets:

- **Best Foods**

- **Low-Carb Diets Better for Controlling Blood Pressure**

Here are links to information about the Glycemic Index and its more helpful but neglected smarter cousin, the Glycemic Load:

- **Wikipedia Entry on Glycemic Load**

- **Glycemic Index and Glycemic Load for 100+ foods**

****

The twelve rules above give you a complete, comprehensive diet and maintenance plan in less than 1,000 words. Not bad, considering that you could go to Amazon and spend 1,000 dollars on diet books and not learn anything important that is not covered in my 1,000-word program. It's small enough to print it out and put on your refrigerator.

Your first inclination may be to carefully count the calories you eat. Unfortunately, that's a terrible idea. Calorie counting is a mess, and the experts who say things like "You need to jog for forty miles to burn off the calories in the Hershey's Kiss that you just snuck into your mouth" are flipping idiots. Calorie counting is almost impossible, and not as important as you might think.

ৡ৾ঌৡ৾ঌৡ৾ঌ

Do Calories Count? The Surprising Answer

Calories count. A lot. However, a calorie is *not* a calorie. Calories from different foods are metabolized differently, with different results. Worse, calorie counts often have little to do with the number of calories we absorb. Dieters, diabetics, etc. are monitoring their calories based on inaccurate, obsolete information: the calorie counts and the available grams of sugar are simply wrong.

Calorie counting is a mess.

In *Scientific American*, Rob Dunn focuses on three issues:

- Almost every packaged food features calorie counts on its label. Most counts are inaccurate because they are based on a system of averages that ignores the complexity of digestion.

- Recent research reveals that how many calories we extract from food depends on which species we eat, how we prepare our food, which bacteria are in our gut and how much energy we use to digest different foods.

- Current calorie counts do not consider any of these factors. Digestion is so intricate that calorie counts may never be accurate.

Calorie Counts Are Wrong – and Not Getting Better

Counting calories seems easy. A calorie (kilocalorie to purists) is a measurement of heat: it is the amount of heat required to raise one kilogram of water (2.2 lbs.) by one degree Celsius (1.8 degrees Fahrenheit). Fats provide approximately nine calories per gram, alcohol has seven, and carbohydrates and proteins deliver just four. Every nutrition label, every diet book, and every fitness tracker relies on these numbers, which were developed in 1896 by American chemist Wilbur Olin Atwater.

However, Atwater was trying to estimate the average number of calories in one gram of fat, protein, and carbohydrates, not in actual foods. The problem: no two foods are the same; they are all digested differently. Think about corn oil and corn. If you sprinkle corn oil on a salad, then 100% of that oil will be available to your body as soon as it hits your small intestines, and little work will be required to digest it.

Now, think about an ear of corn. There's some oil and a lot of carbohydrate in each kernel, but both require processing Your teeth chew and mash the kernels, your stomach grinds and breaks up the mash with powerful acids, enzymes, etc., and then your intestines take over. It will be many hours before the last nutrients are extracted, and even then many kernels will remain intact after they are eliminated. Finally, your body will have expended an unknown number of calories to process the corn that is absorbed and the corn that is eliminated.

It is possible to estimate the calories in the corn oil in a salad, but impossible to estimate the calories available to different people from the same ear of corn.

Calorie Counting: A Riddle Wrapped in a Mystery Inside a Doughnut

And it gets worse. Young plants have relatively thin cell walls, so breaking them down during digestion is easy. However, older plants have sturdier cell walls and are harder to digest. The result: we extract fewer net calories from older plants than from young ones.

There's no way to estimate the age of the different fruits, vegetables, and grains that we buy and no way to estimate how our bodies will digest them. As a result, there's no way to accurately estimate how many calories we will absorb from them, or how many calories we use to digest them.

Calorie counts are at best estimates. And now it gets even more complicated.

Your body is unique. It has a unique digestive process and a unique assortment of gut bacteria. If you and I were given identical portions of food, we would extract a different net number of calories. In the case of pure sugar or pure oil, the differences would be slight. We would both extract most of the available calories.

However, real food is very different from pure sugar and pure oil. If you and I were given identical meals of wild venison and a salad with seeds and nuts, our bodies would react very differently. Venison is tough and stringy; seeds have hard cellulose shells designed to pass through the intestines intact so that they can sprout and grow in a friendly pile of dung. Venison, seeds, and nuts all require a great deal of chewing, an hour or so of mashing in the stomach's acid bath, and then more hours of processing in the small intestines, where natural enzymes and gut bacteria break down the mash into digestible components. Our bodies are different; our digestive processes will be different, and the results will be different.

And now it gets even more complicated.

I don't eat meat, so I don't have healthy colonies of meat-loving bacteria. If you are a meat-eater, you do. On the other hand, my tree-hugging bugs are experts at breaking down seeds and nuts. As a result, we could eat identical plates of food but absorb very different amounts of calories and nutrients, and expend very different amounts of energy in the process. If we both ate exactly 500 calories of food, you might absorb a net of 400 calories and I might absorb 300. Or vice versa. No one can say. That's why the calorie counters from your Fitbit or sites like www.myfitnesspal.com are only slightly better than the advice from your friendly local astrologer.

A Calorie Is Not a Calorie

So... a calorie is not a calorie. What counts is the source. Not surprisingly, this hasn't stopped Big Food from lying about it. Here's a quote from a book my wife and I use frequently, The Fat Chance Cookbook, by Dr. Robert Lustig and my friend, Chef Cindy Gershen:

The Coca-Cola Company's 2013 video "Coming together" states, "Beating obesity will take action from all of us, based on one simple common-sense fact: all calories count, no matter where they come from, including Coca-Cola and everything else with calories..." In other words, "A calorie is a calorie."

What nonsense.

Lustig and Gershen nail it: Coca Cola (and all sugary drinks) provide a textbook definition of empty calories. Sodas and sports drinks have sugar, an assortment of artificial additives, and sometimes a meaningless sprinkling of micro-nutrients to impress poorly informed health nuts. They do not have nutritive value, so if someone drinks 1,500 calories of Coke every day (easy to do) he will still need additional 2,000+ calories from real food with real nutrients. All those empty Coke calories will make him fat and diabetic.

If he hadn't swilled all that Coke, he would be less hungry, not more. Why? Because despite what we have been told by the sanctimonious-sounding, sociopathic sleezeballs who write advertising copy for Coca Cola, a calorie is not a calorie.

What Is the Solution?

Since published calorie counts are, at best, educated guesswork, how can you design a program that includes sufficient nutrition but not too many calories? Amanda Clark's system works; it's a bit pricey but worth the money. Dr. Robert Lustig and Chef Cindy Gershen have an excellent solution in their book *The Fat Chance Cookbook*. If you know about others, write to me: jay@weightzonefactor.com and I'll blog about them. Clark and Gershen are my friends and I'm happy to recommend their work, but there are other good programs. (Note: it may seem strange that this diet book recommends other diets. Not strange at all. No book has all of the answers – certainly this one doesn't.)

In general, instead of counting calories, stick with The 16 Words. Okay – the first twelve words: "Eat reasonable portions of fresh, healthy foods" and "Avoid processed foods and sugars." If you want to lose weight, have the minimum amount of foods that keeps you from getting sudden hunger attacks, and you will be fine.

Calories aren't the enemy; hunger is.

****

Dr. Lustig believes that the main factor driving the modern obesity epidemic is an excess of sugar – specifically, fructose – in our diets. However, many people point to gluten, a protein found in wheat and a few other grains that allows dough to rise. Is gluten a major contributor to the obesity crisis?

৵৵৵৵৵

Will a Gluten-Free Diet Help You Lose Weight?

People used to fear saturated fat. Patients with three days to live wouldn't eat saturated fat because it might give them heart disease in 2047. Pet lovers wouldn't feed saturated fat to their dogs, even though it's good for dogs. Which brings me to gluten (somehow).

Gluten is the third food to be demonized in my lifetime. In the Fifties and Sixties, salt became the Great Satan, guilty of raising the blood pressure of every living thing from human beings to slime mold. Then, in the Eighties and Nineties, the evils of salt faded as saturated fat became The Prince of Darkness – the cause of heart attacks in human beings, dung beetles, and all of their relatives. Apparently, we need some evil food that we can point to and say, "There! That's the reason I'm unhealthy."

Gluten: The Latest Fear-Food

During the last few years, as researchers found that saturated fat is not as dangerous as they thought, gluten became the latest fear-food. However, very few people know what it is. (Gluten is a composite of two proteins that allows bread to rise.) Found in wheat, barley, and rye, it gradually damages the intestines of people with celiac disease, an autoimmune disease.

Celiac disease prevents the absorption of many nutrients and sets off a slew of related health problems, which can include anemia, osteoporosis, fatigue, and more. Celiac disease is miserable, if you have it.

The good news is that you probably don't. Less than 1% of us do. However, another 5% or so have a related and poorly understood condition known as non-celiac gluten intolerance (NCGI). They don't have celiac disease, but they cannot tolerate gluten. That means about 6 people in 100 cannot eat foods that have gluten. The other 94% of us can. So naturally, half the country has begun to avoid gluten the way I avoid spiders.

According to CNN, more than one-third of American adults are consciously avoiding gluten, even though few of them need to. However, many of these people report that they feel better and have lost weight. How can that be? Millions of people cannot be wrong.

The explanation is both simple and obvious, even though CNN missed it. (Sanjay Gupta: call me.) No one goes on a gluten-free diet; they go on a wheat-free diet. (Celiac patients being professionally treated are an exception.) If you switch from having eggs and toast for breakfast to having eggs and fruit, you will consume fewer calories and more nutrition, and you may be less hungry at coffee break.

You may wonder, "What is wrong with a little whole wheat toast?" Nothing, if you can tolerate it. However, from massive anecdotal evidence, it is clear that many people cannot, even though they do not have celiac disease. They feel better and lose weight when they eliminate wheat from their diets. And people who go on gluten-free diets eliminate wheat.

Gluten-Free Diets Are Making People Fat

Such a simple story could not be allowed to last – the business opportunities were too great. What we are seeing today is a repeat of the fat-free craze that ramped up in the Eighties, a craze that caused more heart attacks than gelato ever did. Today, more than a third of American adults are obese, and gluten-free products are growing more rapidly than fat-free foods did thirty years ago. Betty Crocker has gluten-free brownie mix, Pillsbury has gluten-free pizza crust, General Mills has gluten-free cereal, and Tyson has gluten-free bacon. (Apparently, many Tyson customers believe that the average pig has gluten growing somewhere in its ass.)

Manufacturers have not tried to maintain reasonable levels of nutrients in gluten-free processed foods. They simply produce junk that tastes good. The result: people who were losing weight by avoiding grains are now eating gluten-free processed foods and gaining weight again. That has probably happened to many of the people reading this.

And what about you? Should you avoid gluten? Maybe. Ask your gastroenterologist. If the answer is yes, avoid food made with wheat, rye, and barley, read labels, and avoid processed food even if it claims to be gluten-free. The Mayo Clinic has an easy-to-understand gluten-free diet. However, diets that are truly gluten-free are almost impossible to maintain for very long – gluten is everywhere.

If you want to lose weight and think that avoiding grains will help, don't go on a gluten-free diet unless your doctor recommends it. Jay's Perfect Protein-Centered Diet is a better choice. It's much easier to stick with and you may lose weight more rapidly.

That's the good news for your health. The bad news is ten years from now, if the gluten-free craze continues, the world will be fatter than ever.

Additional Reading:
What is Gluten?
What Is Celiac Disease?
The Gluten-Free Craze – **Is It Healthy?**
Five Myths About Gluten

ৡ৵ৡ৵ৡ৵ৡ৵ৡ৵

Will the Paleo Diet Help You Lose Weight?

Paleo, the most popular diet of the decade, sounds simple: if you eat the way our cavemen ancestors did, you'll lose weight and be healthier. Just one problem: no one knows what cavemen ate. The people who created the Paleo Diet guessed, and they were wrong. How do we know? By studying the fiber in Paleo Poop.

What is a Paleo Diet?

People on a Paleo diet eat fruits, vegetables, lean meats (preferably grass-fed or wild), seafood, nuts and seeds, and healthy oils. They avoid grains, dairy, processed foods and sugars, legumes, starches, and alcohol. However, at least two major changes have occurred since the Paleolithic days:

- Modern humans eat just a small fraction of the fiber that our ancestors ate.

- Our gut bacteria have changed dramatically.

If you want to diet successfully, you'll need to account for both of these changes.

How Did the Paleo Movement Start?

Paleo doesn't account for any of these changes, but we can. Let's build a better Paleo Diet based on what scientists have learned in the thirty years since S. Boyd Eaton and Melvin Konner wrote the article that touched off the Paleo movement. (Yes, that was an intentional Paleo Poop Pun. There might be more.)

The authors reasoned that our digestive process has been shaped by several hundred thousand years as hunter-gatherers, not by the brief 10,000-year span since the advent of farming. Meat, probably lots of it, as well as fruits and vegetables were Paleo-friendly. The staples of agriculture – breads, grains, dairy, starches, legumes, and alcohol – were not. Processed foods and refined sugars – very modern inventions – were also excluded.

However, the authors' basic assumptions about what our ancestors ate and what has changed since then were wrong. This doesn't mean that the Paleo Diet doesn't work; it is spectacularly successful for those few people who (A) adhere to its stringent rules and (B) center their diets on fruits and vegetables, not protein. However, this Spartan regimen is unnecessary.

Paleolithic cavemen were humans. They weren't quite Homo Sapiens, but (like members of Congress) they were close. And cavemen were smart, resourceful omnivores: they ate whatever they could find (again, like members of Congress). If they found a carcass brought down by a large predator such as a lion or bear, and if the carcass was near a fruit tree, the cave family would feast on meat and fruit – and fat, and bone marrow. Unappealing, but surprisingly healthy.

If there wasn't a convenient carcass to scavenge or a slow-moving animal to kill, and if there were no fruit trees to shake, our ancestors ate whatever they could find: <u>tubers</u>, roots, and wild plants of every variety.

True Paleo Diets Are Not Possible in the Modern World

Modern humans can live and thrive on a "Paleo Diet"; however, they will be living a pseudo-Paleo lifestyle and eating pseudo-Paleo foods. The foods that were available to our ancestors are no longer available to us. The plants are different, the nutrients they contain are different, and our populations of gut bacteria have evolved accordingly.

Let's assume that you want to live the Paleo lifestyle but do not want to move to the Amazon rainforest and become a hunter-gatherer. Very reasonable. However, you are going to have to purchase your Paleo foods from a decidedly un-Paleo supermarket. At first, shopping will seem easy and healthy; not purchasing processed foods is a terrific start. But you'll quickly get into trouble: supermarkets do not have any true Paleo foods. None. If you are a dedicated Paleo Puppy but live in a city, you'll need to become an urban forager and live on coconuts and road kill.

Food has evolved and our gut bacteria have evolved. They are often inferior, compared with both our Paleo ancestors and with modern hunter-gatherer societies. (Yes, hunter-gatherers still exist in the Amazon and elsewhere.) Produce is different, and the meat at the local supermarket comes from poor animals that have spent most of their lives confined to tiny spaces. It has little in common with the wild game we evolved to hunt or scavenge.

How do we know this? By studying fossilized human feces.

Paleo Poop Is Research Gold

Researchers analyzing human coprolites (fossilized paleo poop) have discovered that our foraging ancestors literally ate ten times as much fiber as we do. Skins, husks, seeds and stems – our ancestors ate remarkable amounts of unprocessed produce. The produce contained vast amounts of both soluble and insoluble fiber, which dramatically improved their entire digestive process.

Fiber was a major part of our ancestors' diets, but few modern humans get enough. Everyone worries about getting the right proportions of the three basic macronutrients – protein, fats, and carbohydrates – but few people realize that fiber is a fourth, quasi-macronutrient. We do not use it for calories or energy, of course, but that is its main value: it slows down and modulates the digestion of other nutrients as they travel through the intestines, so that the body can absorb and use them more efficiently.

Of equal importance, fiber encourages the growth of healthy colonies of gut bacteria – bacteria that promote healthier digestion and help prevent obesity.

Fiber slows down the absorption of sugar, which is essential for good health. When our Paleo ancestors were stomping around, this carefully regulated absorption of sugar kept them alive and healthy. It allowed their bodies to store some sugar for immediate energy and to store the rest as fat, for future periods of starvation. Unfortunately, in the modern world, where apples have been replaced by apple juice and bananas by banana daiquiris, a diet high in refined sugars can overload the pancreas and ultimately cause Type II diabetes.

Smarter Paleo: Eat More Fiber, Not Just More Meat

First, the bad news. You can't simply take fiber supplements or fiber-enhanced processed foods; that will help your bowel function but not your pancreas.

Now, the good news. To strengthen your insulin mechanism, improve digestion and lose weight, you simply need to eat a variety of produce with most meals – unpeeled, unprocessed, and pretty much unchanged from how it was harvested. Yes, this is boring advice, not a miracle cure, but it works. Miracle cures never do.

Too many Paleo people try to diet by eating massive portions of meat – often fatty meat. Wrong. They should eat massive quantities of fiber and reasonable portions of healthy protein with most meals. (Why 'most meals', not 'every meal'? No one is perfect.)

A plant-based, protein-centric program that includes legumes, dairy, and whole grains (not just whole grain flour) is healthy. Moreover, it is not the same as merely adding a few fruits and veggies to an old-fashioned Atkins diet, which is what most Paleo adherents do.

By now you have noticed that I often disparage gimmicky diets that promise magic weight loss solutions. Gimmicks are never successful, long-term; hard work and a plan usually are. The Paleo Diet, as sold to us in books, articles, lectures, protein supplements, etc., is a gimmick. Part truth, part macho chest-beating fantasy. However, if you keep the valuable parts (center most of your meals around a protein) and ignore the hype and conjecture (fruit is unhealthy), you can develop a diet that you can live with for life.

Additional Reading:

Insights from Characterizing Extinct Human Gut Microbiomes

Study of Hunter-Gatherers' Guts Reveals Ancient Microbes

What Discovery of Oldest Human Poop Reveals About Neanderthals' Diet

How to Really Eat Like a Hunter-Gatherer: Why the Paleo Diet Is Half-Baked by Ferris Jabr

Paleo fantasy, by Marlene Zuk

కా కా కా కా కా

Why Fruit Is Safe on a Low-Carb Diet

Here's a fact few diet 'experts' know: low-carb dieters can eat fruit. Fruit and its sugars will not stop you from losing weight.

I know – for years you've been told that to diet successfully, you must spend months eating nothing but protein and vegetables. Who invented that law? A fat prison warden?

Let's put a little rationality into low-carb living. First, use the three 16-Word Diet rules, not Diet Prison rules. On the topic of fruit, 16-WD says: (1) Eat reasonable portions of fresh, healthy foods, and (2) Avoid processed foods and sugars.

Fresh, whole fruit passes both tests. Also, if you are watching your carbs, the carbs will not slow down your weight loss. Here's why:

The Carbohydrate Problem

The problem with carbs is their effect on your blood sugar. After you eat, say, a bag of M&M's or six slices of white bread, your blood sugar can go up and down faster than your Congressman's underwear. If you overload on sugar occasionally, relax: life is short and you should enjoy it. However, if you overload on sugar as part of a lifestyle, there is a strong chance that you will develop Type 2 Diabetes. Nothing sweet is as good as diabetes is bad.

But you know this already. And you also know that foods containing too much refined sugar or refined grains are the worst. Those carbs are absorbed into your bloodstream at hyperspeed and they will quickly overload your pancreas and liver. Fruit is essentially a pretty little sack of sugar and water, which is why every low-carb maven tells you that fruit is bad for your diet. And every low-carb maven is wrong. Fruit juice is bad for you, canned fruit is bad for you, but raw fruit is fine.

Why? Because what counts is not the number of grams of carbs that you eat, but how fast those carbs hit your bloodstream. If you drink fruit juice, a massive sugar overload will be absorbed into your bloodstream in a very short time, and a cascade of disastrous events often follows. But raw fruit is different. When you eat it, the sugar is absorbed slowly, over the course of hours, and some is never absorbed at all.

Why Fruit Is a Safe Source of Carbs

Natural fruit sugar is stored inside cell walls made of cellulose, and those walls are tough to break open. Some sugars are released when you chew, some are released as your stomach grinds and mashes away, and some are released in your small intestine. The entire digestive process takes up to twenty-four hours, so there's never an overload. And one last, unpleasant but necessary detail: a significant percentage of fruit sugar is never absorbed. The cell walls are never broken down, and the glucose and fructose they protect pass through your body undigested. Think about corn. Now stop.

That's why fruit is fine on a low-carb diet. The fruit sugars (glucose and fructose) are absorbed gradually, the way they should be. They won't overload your pancreas and they won't hurt your diet (unless you eat too much). How much is too much? Everybody (and every body) is different. Use common sense and eat reasonable portions. That's why this program is called Dieting for Adults.

How Many Carb Grams Per Day Are Safe?

Many books and articles eliminate fruit altogether, so that low-carb dieters can stay below a specific number of grams of carbs per day. 150 and 60 are the most popular limits, even though both numbers were chosen at random – they are arbitrary and meaningless. Think about this: if you are told to stay below 150 grams of carbs per day but you eat 151 grams of carbs, have you broken your diet? Also, ask yourself my favorite question: why would any sound diet advice apply equally to a sedentary grandmother and to her grandson, the football player?

A research study published in the *British Medical Journal* concluded that fruit can safely be eaten by people at risk for Type 2 Diabetes. Here is a quote from the abstract: "Greater consumption of specific whole fruits, particularly blueberries, grapes, and apples, is significantly associated with a lower risk of Type 2 Diabetes, whereas greater consumption of fruit juice is associated with a higher risk."

A final thought: a surprising new study from the Department of Nutrition of The Norwich Medical School in the United Kingdom indicates that simply eating fruit, especially fruit high in antioxidants, can prevent or relieve ED in a small but significant number of men.

Men who ate more fruit than average had a 14% reduced risk of having ED. Also, those who ate diets high in the highest antioxidant-rich fruits – including strawberries, blueberries, apples/pears and citrus fruits – had an even greater reduction in ED risk: 19%.

"We already knew that intake of certain foods high in flavonoids may reduce the risk of conditions including diabetes and cardiovascular disease," said study researcher Aedin Cassidy, as quoted by Alice G. Walton in *Forbes*. "This is the first study to look at the association between flavonoids and erectile dysfunction, which affects up to half of all middle-aged and older men." (Note that red wine has high levels of flavonoids, but men who drink two or more ounces of alcohol per day have very high levels of ED. Stick with fresh grapes.)

How valid is the Norwich study? I can't say. First, it wasn't conducted under controlled conditions – that wouldn't be possible. It was based on data gleaned from questionnaires asking men about their eating and exercise patterns for the previous four years. Are memory-based estimations reliable? Tell me – could you accurately estimate how many pieces of fruit you ate daily during the last four years? I can accurately estimate how often I've climbed Mount Everest solo or slept in an igloo with Jennifer Lawrence, but not much else.

Second, the men studied were high-income, middle-aged, white medical professionals – men who tend to be more health-conscious than average. If they also eat fruit regularly, they probably have healthy lifestyles based on smart eating patterns and vigorous exercise, which is the best way to prevent, postpone, or even reverse ED.

Third (and worst), the questionnaires asked men how often they had experienced ED during the previous four years. The average guy has a much better chance of building that igloo and sleeping in it with Jennifer Lawrence than accurately remembering and reporting how often he experienced ED.

Regardless, it's fun to talk about over dinner.

৯৯৯৯৯

Do Any of the Diet Pills Sold Online Work?

Just as there are no magic cures for ED, there are no magic cures for obesity. You cannot go to a health food store or some website you heard about from the checker at Walmart and purchase a diet pill that works. Sorry.

As an hilarious example, here is a strange story about all of the miracle herbal diet pills that have become popular in the last few years: Garcinia Cambogia, Green Coffee Bean Extract, Raspberry Ketones, Açai Berry Extract, Saffron Extract, Proactol Pills, Yacon Syrup, African Mangos, HCG, and LipoSlim. They all have something in common with sexy Samantha Barston, the News 6 Health and Diet reporter who has written about them.

What's the connection? They are all fakes. The diet pills do not work and sexy Samantha Barston does not exist. Regardless, the pills are available all over the Internet, along with her reporting. And yes, people believe her 'recommendations' and spend hundreds of millions of dollars on valueless pills. Attention FDA: are you listening?

I didn't think so.

People frequently write and ask my opinion about some new, magic diet pill they found online. I always evaluate the scientific literature before answering, then give the same response: the new magic diet pill does not work. But recently, I remembered something odd: several of the websites I had visited in the past few months featured attractive female news reporters who had tested the pills and claimed to have lost 25 pounds in four weeks. The same weight loss, different diet pills. Hmmm... I returned to a few sites and found identical claims with identical wording:

"**News 6** reporter **Samantha Barston** loses 25 lbs. on Garcinia Cambogia diet."

"**News 6** reporter **Samantha Barston** loses 25 lbs. on açaí berry diet."

"**News 6** reporter **Samantha Barston** loses 25 lbs. on green coffee extract diet."

No, I am not making this up. Google it.

Who Is Samantha Barston and How Fat Was She When She Started Dieting?

I Googled "Samantha Barston News 6" and found her name with the same picture on countless websites – well-designed sites that would fool anyone who didn't already suspect fraud. I stopped looking after I found ten different sites, each pushing a different product, and each proudly proclaiming that Samantha Barston had tested their Magic in a Bottle and lost 25 pounds (11.4 kg). Apparently, sexy News 6 reporter Samantha had been 250 pounds (113.6 kg) *overweight* before she started taking her first diet pill. Who hired her? Chris Christie?

(Note: The picture shown on every site is of Melissa Theuriau, a real French journalist who was voted one of the most beautiful TV reporters in the world. That research was fun.)

It got worse. There is no significant research behind any of these supplements. A few studies exist, but they are very small, poorly done, or outright frauds. Also, the websites offer no way to contact the site managers – a strong sign that the site is hiding something or that the site operators are themselves hiding. A few offer links that go to parent sites, but the parent sites are in China and the site is written in Chinese characters. Health supplements made in China and sold over-the-counter, without regulation. How... appetizing.

Again, here is a partial list of diet products recommended by Samantha Barston (and Dr. Oz) that do not work: Garcinia Cambogia, Green Coffee Bean Extract, Raspberry Ketones, Açai Berry Extract, Saffron Extract, Proactol Pills, Yacon Syrup, African Mangos, HCG, and LipoSlim. If you are buying any of the products on that list, then you are swallowing capsules of crud that may have been manufactured in an unregulated, unsupervised factory in China. In China, where they put antifreeze in baby formula and where the dog food kills dogs. Do you want to lose weight that desperately?

I didn't think so.

****

Summary

This chapter had an obvious theme: It's fairly easy to design a diet that is healthy and that you can stick with, but it's even easier to get trapped by gimmicky fad diets that offer instant gratification. Next, we'll look at some fad foods that have the same pitfalls.

Chapter 5: We Eat the Wrong Foods; We Avoid the Wrong Foods

Growing up, things were so simple. Mom said "Eat your steak! It's good for you!" and we listened. Then, in the Eighties, low-fat diets became the rage and we lived on chicken breasts – nature's Styrofoam. And then, low-carb staged a comeback and so did fat – all fats. And then there was a limited list of healthy fats – most fats were again Evil Cardiac Killers. And then the list of fats that were healthy to eat began to expand, slowly at first, and then exponentially, until people on the fringe began touting the benefits of extreme low-carb lifestyles, beginning with the Paleo Diet and ending with putting butter in their coffee instead of fat-free milk. (Yes, I'm serious. No, <u>you shouldn't do that.</u>)

This chapter looks at what I call Fad Food Fears: how to spot them and how to avoid them. It isn't easy, but the advice is always the same: go with the best science. Sometimes that is simple to do (there is no scientific evidence supporting the myth that we should drink eight glasses of water a day), but sometimes it is complicated. (Smart people have reasonable-sounding arguments about the dangers of eating GMO foods, but equally smart people point out that we all eat GMO foods every day with no ill effects.) One thing is clear: don't take advice from your friends; that's like taking advice from <u>The Food Babe.</u> My opinion: don't take health advice from anyone who gave herself a nickname that makes her sound like a pole dancer.

There are too many myths surrounding foods for me to cover in a finite book, so let's just look at some of the most popular. And remember this: whenever a friendly website touts an exotic food as being a miracle, the only real miracle is the amount of money they are going to make selling the stuff.

Let's start with a few random comparisons that show you what to look for, and then discuss a few specific foods.

ഏ•ഏ•ഏ•ഏ•ഏ

Some Foods and Additives Are Worse Than Others. Here's How You Can Tell.

Which is worse:

- High fructose corn syrup or MSG?

- Insecticides and fertilizers in non-organic fruits and vegetables, or antibiotics in beef and poultry?

- Food grown or processed in China, or fast foods?

- GMO foods or anything The Food Babe decides she doesn't like?

Eating used to be simple, not frightening. We had cereal for breakfast, PBJ for lunch, meat and potatoes for dinner, dessert if we did our homework. But not anymore. These days we have a wide variety of choices, but most are loaded with sugar, salt, quasi-mysterious additives, chemicals manufactured in giant steel vats, and worse. Half the people in the country refuse to eat food made by the other half.

If you are worried about some food or additive, ask yourself a simple question: 'Is the fear legitimate?' Then, let common sense guide you. Let's look at some additives we love to hate. Which is worse:

High Fructose Corn Syrup (HFCS) or Monosodium Glutamate (MSG)?
Everyone knows that too much MSG gives some people Chinese Food Syndrome. However, everyone is wrong. MSG is not a problem; it is simply an old Food Fear Fad. MSG occurs naturally in a wide variety of everyday foods, such as tomatoes, cheese, tofu, sausages, yogurt, etc. Do you enjoy pepperoni pizza? It's loaded with natural MSG.

Researchers have conducted many double-blind tests; no one has a negative reaction to MSG. People who are positive they have 'Chinese food Syndrome' cannot tell the difference between swallowing MSG and swallowing a placebo. I once shared sushi rolls with a friend who said she had stopped eating Chinese food because MSG made her throat swell up. Sushi rolls and soy sauce both contain high levels of MSG; she was fine. Why? Because no one told her that she was eating MSG. Her fears were groundless.

On the other hand, surprisingly few people have heard of HFCS and fewer avoid it. However, to every independent food researcher I've found, HFCS is unhealthy. Some experts swear it is the unhealthiest sugar on the market; others believe that it is no worse than any other sugar. Either way, HFCS is pure sugar, and pure sugar is pure poison. If HFCS is an ingredient, why buy the food? That's a legitimate fear.

Insecticides and fertilizers in non-organic fruits and vegetables, or antibiotics in beef and poultry?

You may have read articles by famous wellness 'experts' advising people to not eat produce grown from seeds that were treated with insecticides. Why? Because some of the insecticide from the seeds will still be in the plants when you eat them. Sure. Walk through the fresh produce section of your local supermarket and you will inhale more insecticide than that.

The same Food-Fear Mongers also tell us not to eat produce fertilized with anything that didn't come directly from a farm animal. (Manure is organic!) However, the hard scientific evidence against inorganic fertilizers is pretty weak. Trying to avoid them is certainly good for the planet; other than that, save your energy for avoiding foods that are actually dangerous to eat.

For example, most people do not think about the antibiotics being fed to livestock, which is why most people who only buy organic produce happily buy non-organic beef and poultry from the same supermarket. There is almost no chance that fertilizers or insecticides on non-organic produce will hurt you, but there is a small but legitimate chance that the antibiotics in meat will kill you.

Mega-doses of antibiotics are fed to livestock and poultry to prevent disease. It's a smart short-term strategy, but long – term, it is creating drug-resistant superbugs – bacteria that are resistant to all the drugs fed to that cow you just had for dinner. If you catch one of those superbugs, there may not be any antibiotics to save you. How frightening does a little inorganic fertilizer sound now? Fear of meat from animals fed antibiotics is legitimate. It really can 'save the planet'.

Food from China or American Fast Food?

Trick question. Both are potential nightmares. China is one of the most corrupt societies in the world; it over-regulates private lives and under-regulates industry. <u>Chinese food processing plants</u> are a global disgrace, with underpaid inspectors bribed to ignore the under-aged, undertrained children who mishandle the food headed towards your plate. Food production facilities are filthy, sanitation is non-existent, and no one regulates or tests the various chemicals and additives used everywhere.

American fast food is definitely healthier than that; regardless, it is still landfill. You know that fast food is calorie-dense, nutrient-poor, etc. However, have you thought about the people who make it? Scary. If you eat something from McDonald's/Burger King/Taco Bell/KFC/etc., your food was prepared, cooked, and assembled by minimum-wage workers hardly more qualified to handle something edible than those children slaving in Chinese food factories.

Imagine a high school dropout. He's earning minimum wage and working in a hot kitchen frying burgers for eight sweaty hours every day. How concerned about your sanitation will he be? What are the chances that he will bother to wash his hands in the bathroom if no one is watching?

That's why I haven't eaten in McDonald's/Burger King/Taco Bell/KFC/etc. in more than thirty years.

GMO Foods or The Food Babe?

GMO foods are the Grandmother of Food Fear Fads. GMOs (genetically modified organisms) are plants and animals that have undergone some genetic tinkering to give them desirable characteristics. For better or for worse, <u>all of us have been eating GMO Foods</u> for decades, with no ill-effects (soy beans, tomatoes, canola oil, corn, sugar beets, Hawaiian papaya, alfalfa, squash, etc.). Regardless, many smart people worry that GMO foods may contain proteins or other nutrients that could be unsafe to eat. Their fears are overblown; <u>the risk is real but exceedingly low.</u>

It's reasonable for people to refuse to eat GMOs as long as they also refuse to eat: food grown or processed in China, antibiotic-laden beef or poultry from the local supermarket, eggs from farmers who will not let the public see where the chickens are caged, <u>fish farmed in Viet Nam</u>

downstream from open sewers, shrimp farmed in Thailand, and imported-from-anywhere fruits and vegetables treated with unregulated chemicals so that they can survive the long journey to American tables. Compared with every food just mentioned, GMO foods are mother's milk.

Note: I was going to write a few sentences about the deeply unqualified blogger who calls herself The Food Babe but then decided not to bother. How can I take a woman seriously if her nickname makes her sound like a waitress at Hooters? (Yes, I realize that I have taken two cheap shots at her name. However, if you ever read any of the unscientific nonsense she has written, you will understand. Google "Avoid the Food Babe".)

More seriously (for a few sentences), remember the easy test for a food or an additive. Ask yourself, "Is the fear legitimate?" Usually, it turns out to be exaggerated. Remember my Chinese-food-avoiding, sushi-loving friend? Yes, she is a real person, and (surprise!) she only buys organic fruits and vegetables. However, she puts a new flea and tick collar on her dog every month, and the dog sleeps in bed with her. This intelligent woman is worried about micrograms of insecticide on her produce, but she cuddles contentedly with an insecticide-coated Chihuahua.

After writing that last paragraph, I wondered if I do anything similarly ridiculous, and instantly realized that I drink bottled water, not tap, but make tea every morning with tap water. Let's go immediately to the next section.

Additional Reading:
10 Foods You'll Have to Give Up to Avoid Eating GMOs

WebMD: Are GMOs Safe?

ৡ৽ৡ৽ৡ৽

3 Reasons to Stop Worrying About Salt

Salt was the first food additive, and so it was the first chemical that people became unnecessarily afraid of eating. Want to terrify your grandparents? Ask them to pass the salt, then listen to their horror stories. "Your Great Uncle Max put salt on everything he ate and he had three heart attacks and a stroke in the fifth grade!"

It's unhealthy to eat too much salt, right? Wrong. Well, probably wrong. It's very complicated.

Salt: The First Health Food

For centuries, salt was an essential part of life. Used to preserve food for months without refrigeration, salt enabled lengthy travel along trade routes long before the first roads were built, and it allowed settlement in harsh climates – in far northern latitudes, where meat was scarce, and in the hot tropics, where meat quickly rotted.

Prized for its antiseptic qualities, salt was the first health food... until it suddenly wasn't. About a century ago, medical researchers noticed that people who ate large quantities of salt had a high incidence of heart attacks and strokes. They eventually traced down the sequence of events; the sodium in salt caused increased water retention in many people. That caused high blood pressure, which caused all the damage. Water retention (edema) can be deadly.

Salt: The First Unhealthy Food

For more than fifty years, the message spread: salt is a killer and it should be eliminated from everyone's diet. Doctors wrote countless look-alike paperbacks: Killer Salt, Salt Kills, Salt: Black America's Silent Killer, even two books with the same title: Salt, the Forgotten Killer (by Michael Jacobsen), and Salt, the Forgotten Killer (by Dr. Karen Wolfe).

Various organizations came out with recommendations for salt intake; however, they didn't bother to confer with each other, and their recommendations disagreed completely. The American Heart Association set daily dietary sodium targets 'between 1,500 and 2,300 milligrams or lower', despite two inconvenient facts: (1) the target is almost impossible to achieve unless you are a zoo animal in a cage, and (2) there is zero evidence that healthy people will be helped by it.

On the other hand, a report from the Institute of Medicine, which advises Congress on health issues, found no evidence that cutting sodium intake below 2,300 milligrams reduced risk of cardiovascular disease. Again, 2,300 milligrams. As the wonderful old Paul Simon song goes, One Man's Ceiling Is Another Man's Floor.

To point out the obvious, these arbitrary and conflicting sets of rules were applied to everyone, of every age, every height, every weight, etc. Muscular, sweaty, horny NBA stars and their sedentary, flabby, doomed-to-heart-disease fans are all expected to consume the same amount of salt each day. Sure.

Confused yet? It gets worse. Recently, two studies were published in *The New England Journal of Medicine*, and again, their findings were utterly contradictory. Researchers at the Harvard School of Public Health performed a meta-analysis of 107 previous studies and estimated that globally, there had been 1.65 million deaths from cardiovascular causes in 2010 – deaths that could be attributed to sodium consumption above 2,000 milligrams a day. However, in the same issue, a different group of researchers published a paper claiming that people who consumed less than 3,000 mg a day (and people who consumed more than 6,000 mg a day) had an increased risk of cardiovascular events and mortality. People in the 3,000-6,000 mg range had the lowest number of heart-related events.

Salt Researchers Don't Know How to Conduct Good Research

Let's stop here. The different studies of salt consumption are wildly inconclusive, in significant part because the tests were poorly constructed. One major study estimated salt consumption by testing a single urine sample from people and then following them for the next 3.7 years. They were never tested again. Do the results of a single urine sample matter? Not unless you are Lance Armstrong. What matters in the real world is the food you eat and your level of regular, vigorous exercise – not meaningless milligrams of isolated chemical elements, *your lifestyle.*

People who consume high levels of salt usually get most of their calories from processed foods: frozen dinners, canned goods, pre-packaged items, deli meats, pizza, and restaurant meals – items that are inexpensive, easy to prepare, and overloaded with sodium. These consumers are living an unhealthy lifestyle, and they are not likely to avoid sugar or to get much exercise. Sound familiar? For most healthy people, *The 16 Words* are the best way to control blood pressure.

I have been unable to find a single study that explains why healthy people with normal blood pressure should worry about salt consumption. Also, I have been unable to find a single study that focused on the lifestyle choices of high salt consumers instead of focusing narrowly on the milligrams of sodium consumed. Were a high percentage of the people in the high-risk group smokers? Drinkers? Sedentary? Did they live on pepperoni pizza and beer? Without this type of information, the studies are useless.

What Should You Do?

Let's summarize:

1. The experts are in complete disagreement about how much salt people should consume.

2. The studies focused on salt intake only and ignored the fact that people have different bodies, different lifestyles, and different health histories.

3. Do you need a #3? The 'experts' are full of... salt.

So what should you do if you think you eat too much salt? Stop stressing. If you have high blood pressure, try to control it with lifestyle changes that include less sodium. Your doctor can help, but only if he treats you, not just your lab results. However, if you don't have high blood pressure, kidney disease, etc., why are you worried? Just follow T16D: eat reasonable portions of fresh, healthy foods and avoid processed foods and sugars. Third, get regular exercise. It will lower your blood pressure, etc. Finally, stay hydrated. Drink enough water to help flush out excess sodium. If you think you are retaining water for more than a few days, see your doctor. And that is all you need to do.

Now, find some other way to horrify your grandparents.

Additional Reading:

Sodium Scare: Salt Influence On Blood Pressure Statistically Insignificant

Salt intake and cardiovascular disease: why are the data inconsistent?

Flawed Study on Sodium from JAMA

Study suggests recommended salt levels could do more harm than good

Are Low-Salt Diets Necessary (or Healthy) for Most People?

જ⊷જ⊷જ⊷જ⊷જ

How Fructose Makes You Fat & How to Avoid It

If salt is overrated as a food we must avoid, fructose is underrated. It is evil. Fructose is rapidly climbing the lengthy list of Delicious Diet-Destroying Foods We Should Avoid. Soon, fructose will join gluten and trans-fats on a shorter list: Delicious Diet-Destroying Food Ingredients We Would Be Happy to Avoid If We Knew What the Hell They Are.

Should you avoid fructose? Sometimes yes, sometimes no.

What Is Fructose?

Fructose, famous for being the primary ingredient in high fructose corn syrup, is a natural sugar that makes fruits (and some vegetables) sweet. If you stick to fruits and vegetables, raw or lightly cooked, you can eat all the fructose you like. Most of it is held inside cell walls and surrounded by a tough coat of cellulose, which breaks down very slowly, so the fructose dribbles out in tiny, harmless doses. Tiny, delicious, harmless doses.

But this is America, where "tiny, delicious, and harmless" isn't a description, it is an invitation – to convert 'tiny' into 'supersized', to convert 'delicious' into 'overwhelming', and 'harmless' into 'deadly'. Why? Profits. Any food that is supersized and overwhelmingly sweet will generate mammoth profits, and when money is being brought to the bank in wheelbarrows, no one cares about the 'deadly' part.

However, fructose can be deadly. It is a major cause of non-alcoholic liver disease, an ugly way to die decades before you should, and it is a major contributor to chronic metabolic disease, which leads to Type 2

Diabetes, heart disease, and stroke. As little as three cans of sugary soda a day can gradually cause irreparable damage to the liver, pancreas, and other organs.

A can of soda has about as much sugar as two apples. However, the sugar in the apples is protected by layers of fiber and it takes hours to digest. By contrast, the sugar in a can of soda hits the intestinal walls like a firehose aimed at a chain link fence. Our bodies weren't designed to handle so much sugar, so fast.

Fructose, a simple sugar, has advantages to processed food manufacturers: it is abundant, cheap, and very sweet – it's twice as sweet as glucose, its slightly less toxic cousin. It's the major component of high fructose corn syrup (HFCS), which is found almost everywhere, from the obvious (fruit juice and desserts) to the surprising (breads, tomato sauce, and low-fat everything).

Food Manufacturers Create a Sugar Addiction

Fructose would not be a problem if manufacturers used reasonable quantities, but they don't. They add mega-doses of pure HFCS to almost every processed food imaginable, including bread, pizza, frozen entrees, deli meats, etc., knowing that the more they add, the more addicts they will hook on their products. I'm serious: sugar is weakly addictive. That's why Alcoholics Anonymous meetings all offer cookies, doughnuts, and candy: sugar reduces the craving for alcohol and other drugs. It isn't heroin, but it stimulates the same pleasure centers in the brain that narcotics and alcohol do. If you keep eating too much of it, sugar will eventually hook you. Your brain and your gut bacteria will both demand it. And the deeper the addiction, the more sugar-laden processed food you will buy.

Want proof? Try to find an obese person who doesn't love and crave sugar. You can't. You will find very heavy people who do not like salty foods, bitter foods, sour foods, fermented foods, etc., but you will rarely find an obese person who doesn't like sugar. Does your obese friend prefer pizza and pretzels? They have more sugar than salt, and the sweetest-tasting sugar is… fructose.

The damage fructose causes is well understood: the liver metabolizes it as if it were alcohol. In fact, by the time fructose hits the liver it has effectively become alcohol, having been transformed by the body in almost the same way that yeast transforms sugary grape juice into wine. A small amount of fructose is stored in the liver (as fat – don't ask), and it gradually weakens the liver's ability to function properly. One result: the pancreas produces too much insulin, but the body doesn't use it properly. The result: weight gain and high blood pressure. As years go by, the effects cascade into diabetes, heart disease, and stroke.

And now things get sticky.

Which Delicious Diet-Destroying Additives should you avoid? Fructose, high fructose corn syrup, both, or all sugars? It's a serious, hotly debated controversy, and the experts are divided into two camps. One side, led by Dr. Robert Lustig, believes that since fructose is destructive to the liver it is worse than glucose, which is essential to every cell of the body. The other side says that the studies are inconclusive and that all carbs are capable of damaging the liver. There's an excellent, non-technical discussion of both sides of the debate in a Big Picture Science podcast – just skip through the first five minutes, which were designed to get slow-witted high school students to stop sexting.

Who Is Right?

Both sides have good science behind them, and while the 'Fructose is the biggest evil' camp seems to be winning, I don't care. Manufacturers of processed foods decide how much sugar to use in their products based on elaborate taste tests and sophisticated sales projections, not by consulting with cardiologists. Asking food manufacturers to decide which sugar is healthier is like asking Hannibal Lecter which is healthier: Girl Scout cookies or Girl Scouts.

The anti-fructose argument is countered by the fact that every sugar additive can make us fat. Any type of added sugar. Fructose may indeed be worse than the rest, but the others are close behind. Also, if you remove additives containing fructose from your diet, every type of added sugar will be gone – table sugar, honey, maple syrup, agave syrup, etc. are all loaded with both fructose and glucose. What's left – fruits, vegetables, proteins, dairy, whole grains (not whole grain flour, *whole grains*), and no processed foods – defines a perfect diet.

(As a side note, you may be eating honey, maple syrup, agave syrup,

Sugar-In-The-Raw, or some other sweetener that you have read is healthier than sugar. Sorry, they are not. Those stories are 100% marketing hype. Yuppie sweeteners may have a few additional minerals or other nutrients, but not enough to nourish your pet turtle. Certainly not enough to nourish you. They are all sugars, and they are all unhealthy.)

What is the best way to sweeten something? Raw fruit, if possible. Coarsely grated apples or carrots are wonderful ways to sweeten baked goods, and they will release most of their sugars slowly, which doesn't affect your pancreas. Coffee and tea taste much better unsweetened than with artificial sweeteners – try it for a week or two.

The only facts that count are these: Refined sugar – every type of refined sugar – is slow-acting poison, and fructose may be the worst. If you want to improve your life, avoid sugar passionately, the way that Hannibal Lecter would avoid tofu burgers. You'll do fine.

Additional Reading:
Fat Chance (Dr. Robert Lustig)
Is Sugar Toxic? (Gary Taubes)
High Fructose Heart Risks
Does Fructose Make Us Crave High-Calorie Foods? Maybe – But It May Not Matter.

৯৶৯৶৯৶

Are Artificial Sweeteners Making You Gain Weight?

If you decide to reduce your sugar consumption, should you use artificial sweeteners? Sweet'N Low, Equal, Splenda, etc.?

Artificial sweeteners are everywhere, from soda to cough syrups. Are they helping us lose weight? Making us fatter? Do they help control diabetes? Are they healthier than sugar or are they poisonous, as several chain emails suggest? Researchers keep asking smart questions; their answers have taught me more about my colon (and yours) than I wanted to know.

Artificial sweeteners and human colons don't often come up in the same sentence, but that is changing. According to an article in *Nature*, sugar substitutes such as Sweet'N Low, Equal, and Splenda (saccharin, aspartame, and sucralose), which are widely used to combat obesity and diabetes, may instead be contributing to the global epidemic of both diseases.

Experiments — first with mice and then with people — show that sugar substitutes can increase blood sugar levels instead of reducing them. It turns out that our intestinal tracts are lined with the same sweet taste receptors as are found on our tongues (which again is more than either of us wanted to know). The problem: artificial sweeteners can stimulate intestinal taste receptors just as merrily as real sugar does, which tricks the body into raising blood sugar levels.

Gut bacteria compound the problem. Sugar substitutes can alter the microbiome, which can trigger higher blood glucose levels — a risk factor for obesity and Type 2 Diabetes. That low-fat, no-sugar-added frozen yogurt you have pretended to enjoy for years hasn't done you any good. Sorry.

Do Sugar Substitutes Affect Our Metabolism?

According to Eran Elinav, a physician and immunologist at Israel's Weizmann Institute of Science who is also the lead author of the study published in *Nature,* "Our discovery is cause for a public reassessment of the massive and unsupervised use of artificial sweeteners." That's a very serious statement about the future of public policy, and it shows that Elinav believes the implications of his findings are extremely serious.

First, his team worked with mice. They found that mice fed saccharin, sucralose, or aspartame developed higher levels of glucose intolerance than did those fed only glucose. However, when the animals were given antibiotics to kill their gut bacteria, glucose intolerance was prevented.

Next, when the researchers transplanted feces from glucose-intolerant, saccharin-fed mice into the guts of healthy mice bred to have sterile intestines, those healthy mice also became glucose-intolerant. The conclusion: the saccharin fed to the first group of mice encouraged the growth of gut microbes that triggered higher levels of blood sugar in both groups.

(Take a moment to sympathize with the poor mice who received the fecal transplants. They spent their entire lives in a cage, and their poop chutes were the frequent targets of poop shoots.)

Fake Sugar, Real Human Trials

After Elinav's team proved their hypothesis with mice, they moved up to people. The question was: did artificial sweeteners make people obese and pre-diabetic, or did obese, pre-diabetic people simply consume more artificial sweeteners than their thinner, healthier friends?

The team recruited seven lean, healthy volunteers who did not normally use sugar substitutes and gave them the maximum acceptable daily dose for a week. Four became glucose-intolerant; their gut microbiomes shifted towards a fairly specific blend of bugs known to increase susceptibility to metabolic diseases. However, the other three seemed resistant to saccharin's effects (at least for seven days). "This underlines the importance of personalized nutrition – not everyone is the same," says Elinav.

"Susceptibility to sweeteners can now be predicted ahead of time by profiling the microbes in people," said Eran Segal, a co-author of the study and also, apparently, of Minority Report. Segal's statement is astonishing. People have felt guilty about their 'sweet tooth' for centuries, but this 'weakness' may simply be the result of chemicals manufactured by bacteria living in their intestines.

On the other hand, people who are naturally thin despite downing Clydesdale-portions of sugar every day have felt superior for centuries, and their only real superiority may be a better collection of gut bacteria. Suddenly, that poop shoot sounds attractive. Wait...

The attraction just faded.

Sweeteners Can Affect Your Brain, too

About a year after the Weizmann Institute study was published, Australian researchers at The University of Sidney found that artificial sweeteners (specifically, sucralose) may cause the brain to send out signals that prompt us to eat more real sugar. In their study, fruit flies ate 30% more calories when their food was artificially sweetened than when it was naturally sweetened. Later, when the researchers gave real sugar to the two groups of flies, they saw differences in how their brains responded. The sucralose-habituated mice had more activity in their brains in response to the real sugar, which suggests that the sugar may have tasted sweeter after the fruit flies had become accustomed to sucralose.

"After chronic exposure to a diet that contained the artificial sweetener sucralose, we saw that animals began eating a lot more," said study author Greg Neely. "Through systematic investigation, we found that inside the brain's reward centers, sweet sensation is integrated with energy content. When sweetness versus energy is out of balance for a period of time, the brain recalibrates and increases total calories consumed."

In other words, when the brain perceives sweetness without calories – the two go together in natural foods – it pushes back. It recalibrates to the strange balance, or imbalance, it's gotten used to. "The pathway we discovered is part of a conserved starvation response that actually makes nutritious food taste better when you are starving," says Neely. The flies also exhibited other "symptoms," like hyperactivity, insomnia and glucose intolerance.

"A similar phenomenon was found when the study was replicated in mice, which suggests that it exists across species, from insect to mammal. And presumably, if it's there in mice it would also be present in humans – at least it's likely to be, given what researchers have seen in humans consuming sweeteners." (Alice G. Walton.)

Should You Cut Out Sugar Substitutes?

The evidence against artificial sweeteners is strong. They may make you hungry; they may make you gain weight; they may make you more prone to Type 2 Diabetes. However, the studies I found were all, like Elinav's, small and short – term. I'm always leery of research conclusions based on such a small sample size. That said, there have been enough studies to convince me that we should be careful.

If you consume a lot of artificial sweeteners – in diet soda, 'sugar-free' products, foods you prepare at home, or in your coffee – there are just two things to do:

1. Cut back on both artificial sweeteners and sugar.

2. Stop whining because you have to cut back on both artificial sweeteners and sugar.

The first rule is easier than the second. If you use two packets in your coffee, try one. If you use one packet, try none. Purchase unsweetened yogurt instead of artificially sweetened yogurt and then add some fruit; the combination of naturally sweet fruit and naturally tart yogurt is a huge improvement over the sweet but flavorless melted plastic glop offered by Dannon, et al. And stop buying diet soda; it's nothing but tap water infused with a witch's brew of frightening chemicals. (If you frequently drink diet soda but insist on buying organic fruits and vegetables, please paste a giant "KICK ME!" sign on your ass.)

You don't need to eliminate sugar substitutes completely, just cut back gradually until they become unimportant. I did this years ago, when the first studies came out. I consumed massive quantities of artificial sweeteners during the years when I weighed over 300 pounds (136 kg); I cut back slowly and never felt deprived. These days, I have a little honey in my first cup of tea every morning, a Diet Coke two or three times a week, and a sugary dessert once or twice a week. I never feel deprived, and you won't, either. Food tastes better when it hasn't been pumped up with sweeteners, real or fake.

The Best Sweetener: Fresh Fruit

Sugar and artificial sweeteners are food additives. One is natural, one is artificial, but both are food additives. You should try to avoid them. Fruit – fresh, unprocessed, unpeeled fruit – is the best possible way to handle your sweet tooth.

No candy in the world is as fragrant and satisfying as a simple, ripe piece of fruit, and unlike candy or dessert, it will not raise your blood sugar. Fruit will also do a great deal to help restore a healthy balance of colonies of gut bacteria, which will make your colon very happy. Just don't write to tell me about it; that is definitely more than I wanted to know.

Additional Reading:

Sugar substitutes linked to obesity

The Bad News About Artificial Sweeteners

Diet Soda Builds Desire, Decreases Satisfaction.

Splenda alters gut microflora and increases intestinal p-glycoprotein and cytochrome p-450 in male rats.

The Evidence Supports Artificial Sweeteners Over Sugar. (Interesting, but note how the author hones in on rare cancers and ignores Type 2 Diabetes.)

ക‑ക‑ക‑ക‑ക

Foods That Can Ruin Any Diet

Salt, sugar, artificial sweeteners, MSG, GMO foods – these are all important food components that you should understand, but they aren't specific foods. Let's briefly look at ten of the most popular foods that people abuse. Later, we'll bore down on a few that will surprise you. But first, a few actual questions I have received:

"Can I eat pancakes on a low-fat diet?" "Can I have Salami and low-carb beer for dinner on a high-protein diet?" "Are fried pork rinds safe?"

I'd give more examples but suddenly I feel queasy. Most people simply do not understand basic facts about dieting and nutrition. Pancakes are saggy, sugary sacks of oily flour, salami is one of the least healthy foods that can be sold without a license, and fried pork rinds are only slightly worse for us than they are for the pig.

Let's look at some of the most common poor choices and see why they can sabotage any diet – low-fat, low-carb, or anything else that is working.

1. AVOID HIGHLY PROCESSED CARBOHYDRATES IN BREAKFAST FOODS. Instant oatmeal, sugary cereals that aren't whole grain, pancakes and French toast (duh), canned fruit, sugar, honey, jelly, and anything marketed to children are miserable. Short-term, you

will be hungry by 11 AM. Long-term, you may develop diabetes or heart disease. Eat these foods on special occasions, not every day.

2.   AVOID PROCESSED FOODS AT LUNCH AND DINNER. They are fast and they taste great. But a commercial kitchen led by a talented chef could make dung beetles taste delicious. Remember that charming image the next time you want a frozen pizza from 7-11.

3.   AVOID PROCESSED MEATS. Sausages, hot dogs, and salami are all baloney. Slimy bags of fat and salt. They also hold a little meat, if you consider snouts and genitals to be meat. If that hasn't convinced you, consider this: The World Health Organizations estimates that people who eat as little as two ounces of processed meats per day increase their chances of colorectal cancer by 18%.

4.   AVOID SUGARY DRINKS. Soda and fruit juices are slow-acting poisons. Soda is water with 10 or more teaspoons of sugar per glass, and some complicated chemicals. Fruit juice is effectively soda with a few minor micro-nutrients; it is missing natural fruit fiber as well as many of the essential phytochemicals, etc. found in whole fruit. Either drink will hit your pancreas like a fire hose aimed at a brick wall: insulin will spray in every direction. First, you'll get a sugar rush and then you'll get hungry. Most of the time, stick with unsweetened coffee, tea, or ice water. Some of the time, relax and drink what you like.

5.   AVOID DESSERTS AND CANDY. These are fine, if only on special occasions. Your birthday is a special occasion. Someone else's birthday is not.

6.   AVOID OR MINIMIZE ALCOHOL. One glass of wine per day is enough for anyone. None is better. Why? Alcohol is a sugar that stimulates the appetite. If you cut just one glass of wine a day, you will cut 175 calories and no nutrients. That's about 64,000 calories per year, plus a reduced appetite. Any questions? And no, alcohol is not guaranteed to protect your heart; the studies have become murky. Any more questions?

7.   AVOID DEEP-FRIED FOODS. Do you really need an explanation?

8.   AVOID FAST FOODS. Ditto.

9.   CHOCOLATE IS NOT ON THIS LIST. Life is too short. Once or twice a month, a little chocolate (or another favorite treat) is terrific. Much more than that and you'll need to cut it out altogether. Your choice.

10. AVOID WHITE FLOUR. In the next chapter, I argue that there's little difference between 100% whole wheat flour and white flour*, yet here I am, contradicting myself. Except I'm not. The two flours have almost identical effects on blood sugar, and the important nutrients in whole wheat flour are easy to get from other foods. However, on a diet you eat less food than is normal, so you need to maximize your intake of every nutrient. Obviously, dieters can avoid grains completely and stay healthy if they eat a variety of fruits and vegetables; however, if you are going to eat bread while dieting, eat the healthiest kinds: 100% whole wheat or 100% whole grain.

If ever you are not sure about how to proceed with a food or a meal, remember this basic advice: **Diet like an adult**. It will never fail you. Think about it the next time you want to buy a bag of fried pork rinds.

ও-ও-ও-ও-ও

Why Whole Wheat Bread Is Not Much Healthier Than White

We all eat bread, but few of us understand basic nutritional facts about it. Here's why: everyone knows that whole wheat bread is healthier than white bread, and everyone is wrong.

There are two traditional reasons to choose whole wheat over white. The small reason: whole wheat flour has important nutrients that have been processed out of white flour. The large reason: white flour makes your blood sugar spike quickly and then crash, whole wheat doesn't. Everyone knows this. Is everyone wrong?

Probably.

On New Year's Eve, 2014, my wife and I had dinner in an extravagant San Francisco restaurant – the kind that makes Disney World look like a non-profit charity. They served freshly baked San Francisco Sour Dough, one of the finest artisanal breads in the country. One of the finest *white* breads. While trying to talk myself into having a second slice (okay, a third), I started thinking about white flour vs. wheat.

Do We Need the Additional Nutrients in Whole Wheat?

If the nutrients processed out of white flour are irreplaceable, how come so many people live healthy, happy lives without consuming any wheat at all? People on gluten-free diets, Atkins, the Paleo Diet, etc., live with little or no wheat and stay healthy, so obviously they do not need the nutrients in whole wheat. That said, what's wrong with a healthy diet that includes white bread?

Easy. Everyone knows that white flour makes your blood sugar spike up and then collapse. But... it doesn't.

An intact kernel (berry) of wheat has three parts: bran, germ, and endosperm. If you eat a whole wheat berry, your teeth will crack it a bit, then your stomach will reduce it to a pasty mess before it travels through your gastrointestinal tract. Some of the nutrients will slowly be absorbed, some will not, and your blood sugar levels will not be affected. Clean and simple. Well, simple.

Flour is different. Particles are vanishingly small: 0.5 to 10 microns. If you put ten or twenty thousand flour particles in a row, your row will be about an inch (2.5 cm) long. Whole wheat flour consists of micron-sized particles of endosperm, bran or germ. White flour particles are mainly endosperm; they have all the carbs but little fiber, vitamins, or other nutrients.

Now, here is the part that most people miss: whether flour is whole wheat or white, each individual particle is pure: pure bran, pure wheat germ, or pure endosperm. When particles of endosperm pass through the intestines, they are quickly converted into glucose, a basic sugar. It doesn't matter if the original flour was whole wheat or white; it is converted and absorbed at the same speed, which means that whole wheat bread and white bread should have identical effects on blood sugar. And as explained above, the bran and wheat germ do not have any nutrients that aren't easily obtainable elsewhere. What's so special about whole wheat? And what is so dangerous about white?

Some Excuses for Eating White Bread Are Legitimate

Anyway, that was my theory over the New Year's Eve dinner table, or at least my excuse for having another slice of sourdough. (It worked.)

But everyone knows that whole wheat bread is healthier than white bread. Every article on nutrition written during the last 50 years says so. So I decided to look for the original studies, to learn why my theory was wrong. I couldn't find any.

I tried Google, and then Bing, and finally <u>PubMed</u>, the best source for original research studies. I did not find a single study showing that the nutrients in whole wheat flour are difficult to obtain from other sources, or that white flour affects blood sugar differently than whole wheat flour does. I did find two small studies from the 1980s, but each one tested fewer than 20 people. Meaningless. I also found an endless list of copycat articles about nutrition claiming that "everyone knows that whole wheat bread is healthier than white bread" ... without proof.

Where's the Proof?

Is it possible that no one has ever proven one of the most popular claims in modern nutrition – one that everyone 'knows' is true?

But wait! How about the Glycemic Index? Doesn't that prove... something? Two points. First, according to <u>Harvard Heath</u>, whole wheat bread and white bread have about the same glycemic index: 71 and 73. Second, the Glycemic Index sucks carbs. It is a miserable metric. <u>According to Wikipedia,</u> it measures how high blood sugar rises in response to eating the specific carbohydrates in specific foods, but not in response to eating the food itself. That's why carrots, a very healthy food on any diet, have a high glycemic index: the sugar in carrot juice is digested rapidly. In real life, most carrot sugar is either digested very slowly, or it passes through the body undigested. Either way, its effect on blood sugar is almost negligible. The Glycemic Index is useless.

The Glycemic Load is a better number, but not by much. Unlike the Glycemic Index, it considers realistic portions of food, so it gives more realistic results. However, both the GI and the GL were computed using just a few test subjects held under strictly controlled, completely unrealistic laboratory conditions. The results have little to do with the real world. And one last thing: the glycemic loads of both types of flour are almost identical – and very low. The effect on your blood sugar is probably the same: identical, and very low.

Conclusions About Whole Wheat vs. White

So here's my surprising conclusion: everyone knows that whole wheat bread is healthier than white bread, and in my opinion, everyone is wrong.

If you are going to eat wheat products, there is no reason to ban white flour. Just follow certain basics:

- Read the ingredient label. Many breads are loaded with sugars, preservatives, and other unnecessary additives. Just like dog biscuits.

- Don't make white flour a major part of your diet – eventually, you will miss the various nutrients that were processed out. This is especially true if you are on a diet. Dieters need all the nutrients they can get and white bread is nothing but empty calories (some of what everyone knows really is true).

- Don't make whole wheat flour a major part of your diet, either. Save room for all of the whole grains: oats, rice, corn, etc. And yes, whole grains are significantly healthier – if grain is a major part of your diet. If you get nothing else from this chapter, remember that sentence. Finally, if you follow a protein-centered program and eat grains just a few times per week, relax and enjoy them – whole or refined.

And if you're lucky enough to get some freshly baked, artisanal San Francisco Sour Dough bread, eat as much as you can, as fast as you can, before someone at your table eats it first. Everyone knows that.

Eight Glasses of Water a Day: Truth, Myth, or Scam?

Now, let's talk about the most important nutrient of all: water. Everyone knows that we have to drink eight glasses of water a day, and once again, everyone is wrong.

These days, when people start strength training or even a simple walking program, they immediately begin to worry about dehydration. And then they start to carry a water bottle around wherever they go, shedding virtuosity all over the rest of us.

The truth is that drinking eight glasses of water a day is great advice if you're a flounder. If you're human, it's a silly health myth that refuses to die. Regardless, dieters obey it like an eleventh commandment: "Thou must drinketh water until thou waketh three times nightly to pee."

Not long ago, I watched Dr. Sanjay Gupta interview some muscular lunk about a diet book he had 'written' in which he shows 'The Best Way to Lose Weight Very Quickly'. (Note: the old 'Lose Weight Quickly' meme is a great way to sell pallet-loads of diet books while helping absolutely no one.) In the interview, Mr. Lunk (that may not be his real name) promoted his theory: people must drink a large glass of water before every meal, and they must drink a great deal more water throughout the day to stay hydrated. To him, eight glasses of water each day was an absolute minimum.

It's a wonderful suggestion if you are racing camels with a band of desert nomads, but not if you are living in, say, Seattle.

Somehow, the hydration myth lingers on, promoted not just by cellophane celebrities but also by solemn, professorial authorities who, with deep gravitas, tell us how important it is to remain hydrated every day. However, before you strap a 64-ounce (1.9 L) water bottle to your hip, remember that the obscure word 'gravitas' was popularized by journalists trying to describe the solemn, professorial authority of Dick Cheney. And think about how that worked out.

Are We All Dehydrated?

Sanjay Gupta is one of the smartest media docs we have. He earned his gravitas legitimately, but during the segment on drinking more water, he said, "We walk around, in our society, chronically dehydrated." Excuse me? You don't need to be a zoologist to know that if there are abundant, safe supplies of water, it is impossible to keep a large group of intelligent mammals dehydrated for more than ten minutes. Evolution weeded out our thirst-ignoring ancestors during The Cambrian Period. And yet, authorities everywhere keep claiming that we do not drink enough water, based on absolutely no evidence at all.

So who created the eight-glasses-of-water-a-day shibboleth? According to Chris Gayomali, in a smart article he wrote for *This Week*, "The very idea of a 'minimal water requirement' is fairly new; it first appeared in dietary guidelines published in 1945 by the Food and Nutrition Board of the National

Academy of Sciences. The academy spuriously suggested that '2,500 ml [2.6 quarts] of fluid should be ingested on a daily basis,' although a primary clinical study was never actually cited." Translation: Someone was guessing. No one knows why.

A Worldwide Scam

The myth lingers, kept alive by organizations such as <u>Hydration for Health.</u> Their advice for health professionals is simple, direct, and has been repeated around the world: "Recommending 1.5 to 2 (quarts) of water daily is the simplest and healthiest hydration advice you can give." However, according to the *British Medical Journal*, "Hydration for Health has a vested interest: it is sponsored by and was created by French food giant Danone, a major producer of bottled water (Evian, etc.)."

The people who gush with effervescent praise over the glories of drinking eight bottles of water a day are the people who sell us bottled water.

And what about the studies saying that hydration is essential for health? Either they were misquoted or they were bad studies. Again from the BMJ, "In 2002, Heinz Valtin published a critique of the evidence in the *American Journal of Physiology*. He concluded that 'Not only is there no scientific evidence that we need to drink that much, but the recommendation could be harmful...' "From the June 2008 *Journal of the American Society of Nephrology,* "There is no clear evidence of benefit from drinking increased amounts of water... There is also no clear evidence of lack of benefit. In fact, there is simply a lack of evidence in general." (2008)

Giant bottled water marketer <u>Danone</u> has taken a popular old myth and turned it into a hugely profitable scam. (FYI, Danone is better known in the US as the maker of Dannon Yogurt.)

Okay. Here's the truth about drinking liquids: If you are a large man playing beach volleyball on a hot, sunny day, drinking eight glasses of water isn't a bad idea. Protect yourself from dehydration. However, if you are a small, slender woman studying for finals in a cool, dark college library, drinking all that water is a terrible idea. At best, you will spend half the day walking back and forth to the toilet. At worst, you will end up in the hospital with <u>water intoxication</u>. That's even less fun than studying for finals in a dark college library.

Obviously, drinking water instead of sugary soda is smart; soda labels should have a skull and crossbones. However, boosting liquid intake for its own sake is useless. It will help improve a few bottom lines; it will not improve your health. On the other hand, despite the widely held notion that tea and coffee dehydrate us, they do not. The minor diuretic effect of caffeine is overwhelmed by the sheer volume of water in a cup of coffee, so if you want to waste your money on a $37 double almond soy latte at Starbucks, don't feel guilty. About the caffeine.

What Rule Should You Follow?

It's very simple: don't let yourself get thirsty. Drink some water, tea, or coffee before you do, especially on hot days or if you are exercising. Don't worry about electrolytes unless you exercise vigorously for more than an hour, spend the day at the beach, etc. And stop stressing over all the rules you are told to follow, including this one.

If you think about it, asking everyone to drink eight glasses of water a day doesn't make any sense. Why should a 5-foot-tall grandmother need to drink the same amount of water as her granddaughter, the 6-foot-tall (183 cm) professional beach volleyball player? Why are eight glasses perfect but not seven or nine? And why is this silly myth still floating about the Internet like a dead flounder?

ৡ৽ৡ৽ৡ৽ৡ৽ৡ৽

Saturated Fat – Were the Experts Wrong Again?

Saturated fat. Everyone knows that it raises cholesterol levels, and everyone knows that it's the root cause of heart attacks and strokes. And yet again, everyone seems to be wrong. Could the real villain be gut bacteria? Do whole milk or perhaps dairy fats in general, long treated as nutritional punching bags, actually improve heart health? The more we learn, the murkier things get.

Two excellent, unrelated articles illustrate the confusion surrounding the once-clear advice about healthy heart habits. First, a paper published in Circulation Research showed the striking percentages by which the wrong mix of intestinal bacteria can raise blood lipid levels (triglycerides and the various forms of cholesterol).

Then, *The Washington Post* published a thoughtful, well-researched article by Peter Whoriskey explaining why saturated fat is not as dangerous as we have been taught, and why foods such as whole milk may actually be beneficial for the heart.

Is Whole Milk a Healthier Choice?

As Whoriskey wrote (I quote him liberally below), the Federal Government's influential Dietary Guidelines for Americans recommends that we "Replace whole milk and full-fat milk products with fat-free or low-fat choices." However, scientists who tallied diet and health records for several thousand patients over a ten-year period found that people who consumed more milk fat had a lower incidence of heart disease.

By warning people against full-fat dairy foods, the United States is "losing a huge opportunity for the prevention of disease," according to Marcia Otto, lead author of several major studies funded by government and academic institutions (and not the dairy industry). "What we have learned over the last decade is that certain foods that are high in fat seem to be beneficial."

Is Saturated Fat the Enemy?

The idea that reducing saturated fat consumption will, all by itself, make people healthier has never been proven. Repeated clinical trials and large-scale observational studies have produced evidence to the contrary; most people who eliminate fats from their diets eat more carbohydrates, especially sugars, and too much sugar is a well-documented cause of heart disease. However, replacing saturated fats with unsaturated fats – found in fish, nuts and vegetable oils – is well known to improve heart health. (This is why the Mediterranean diet is so effective.)

Tufts Dean Dr. Dariush Mozaffarian says that the Federal Dietary Guidelines still cling to the idea that saturated fat from any source is a dietary evil, despite absence of proof. Whole milk is a good example. Fats from dairy appear to have protective effects on the heart and circulatory system that outweigh any negative effects, so why drink skim milk, which is high in carbohydrates and full of additives (read the label). Judging a food solely by how much fat it contains, Mozaffarian said, can too easily blind people to its other benefits. "There's no evidence that the reduction of saturated fats should be a priority."

The Old-Guard Empire Strikes Back...

Many disagree. Penny Kris-Etherton, a nutrition professor at Penn State University and a former member of the Dietary Guidelines advisory committee, says there is "A Mountain of Evidence" explaining how consumption of saturated fats raises the risk of heart disease.

The American Heart Association uses that Mountain as proof that consuming saturated fats raises levels of so-called "bad" cholesterol in the blood, which raises risks of heart disease. The problem is that most of the studies in The Mountain of Evidence were conducted by researchers who went home at night and watched live broadcasts of I Love Lucy. The American Heart Association has a lot of S*l*o*w*-*L*e*a*r*n*e*r*s.

Most research from this century is different. Here are two arbitrary examples:

- In 2013, New Zealand researchers led by Jocelyne R. Benatar collected the results of nine randomized controlled trials on dairy products. They could detect no significant connection between consuming more dairy fat and levels of "bad" cholesterol in the blood.
- Alice Lichtenstein, who served this year on the Dietary Guidelines advisory panel, states, "We have strong evidence that replacing saturated fats with carbohydrates has no effect on cardiovascular disease."

What's going on? Apparently, the source of the saturated fat is important. The saturated fat from dairy seems, on balance, to be protective, but the saturated fat from, say, pork products might be dangerous. Maybe.

... But It Misses Your Gut

One explanation for the conflicting, changing advice might be found in gut bacteria.

We all have thousands of colonies of different bacteria living in our gut. Apparently, some strains are healthier than others. Scientists led by Jingyuan Fu from the University Medical Center at Groningen showed the striking percentages by which your intestinal bacteria can raise your blood lipid levels. Researchers knew that intestinal bacteria can affect lipid levels, but Fu's team was the first to show the sometimes dramatic percentages involved. They found that by factoring in age, gender, genetic factors, and gut microbiome counts, up to 25.9% of HDL variance was explained. They also found that increased microbial diversity was associated with healthy lipid levels.

"Lower gut microbial diversity can now be added as a new risk factor for heart disease." said Fu. Specifically, decreased diversity of gut microbes is strongly associated with high body mass index (BMI) and high triglyceride levels, as well as with a low level of desirable high-density lipoproteins (HDL). In English, if you don't have a broad variety of intestinal bacteria, it will screw up some of your cholesterol numbers. Worse, it can make you fat.

The Simple Defense

How do you increase the diversity of bugs in your intestines? By consistently eating a wide variety of healthy foods, which will encourage a broad variety of healthy bacterial colonies in your digestive tract. The narrower your diet, the fewer strains of bacteria you will support, which makes it easier for the bad ones to take over. Grandma was right again – eat your fruits and vegetables, not just meat and bread.

Commenting on the implications, Dr Fu explained that the microbiome is an interface between diet and drugs. "Fecal transplantation [the process of transplantation of fecal bacteria from a healthy individual into a recipient] has become an attractive intervention for disease prevention and therapy," she noted, in a sentence containing the worst use of the adjective 'attractive' in human history.

Understanding the specific influence that the gut microbiota has on body weight and lipid levels is important, she said, "Because it has implications for how we could control body weight and blood lipid levels through microbiome-targeted interventions."

Which is where we started. We all want to maintain a healthy weight, and to reduce our risk of heart disease and stroke, but we focus on single foods or food groups – either we eliminate them completely or we eat them obsessively. However, the latest research says the best way to stay healthy is to eat reasonable portions of fresh, healthy foods and avoid processed foods and sugars. Hope that sounds familiar...

৯৯৯৯৯

10 Myths about 'Superfoods'

Ever wonder why you never heard of 'superfoods' while you were growing up? Because they didn't exist. Big Agriculture popularized the name to hype the sales of ordinary produce. Their claims about superfoods have something in common with organic fertilizers – both started deep inside a bull. Some superfoods are wonderful choices and some are worthless, but all claim to have magical healing powers – and they don't.

Most 'superfoods' are produced by organic or 'natural' foods companies. The companies have friendly, homespun names, but most are owned by Big Ag. Big Ag now uses the same aggressive techniques to hype superfoods that they used a few years ago to convince us we would all have perfect bikini bodies if we just ate enough SnackWell's.

Didn't work for me.

Let's see which superfoods are really nutritious, and which are just inventive ways to suck money out of your checking account.

1. <u>Kale fights heart disease and cancer:</u> I love kale. It's crunchy, with a sweet peppery flavor. I eat it all the time, in salads and on sandwiches. Kale has important vitamins, minerals, anti-oxidants... you know the story: it's very healthy. However, kale isn't magic. It won't make your hair grow back (I wish!), it won't improve your sex life (I wish harder!!), and it won't do anything other than supply excellent, inexpensive nutrition – like most vegetables. The healthiest thing you can do is to eat a wide variety of fruits and vegetables, very often. And please, do not buy dried kale (or anything else) in pills at the health food store; you may be buying someone's <u>lawn clippings</u>.

2. <u>Quinoa, açaí berries, goji berries, chia seeds, blueberries, Brazil nuts, seaweed, wheat grass, etc. are all Superfoods that you must eat:</u> Did you understand what you just read about Kale being healthy but not having magic powers? Good. You can skip this paragraph. Everyone else: listen carefully. Y*O*U – A*R*E – A – S*L*O*W –L*E*A*R*N*E*R. Let's repeat. Quinoa, açaí berries, goji berries, chia seeds, blueberries, Brazil nuts, seaweed, wheat grass,

etc., are perfectly healthy but they are not magical. You may have heard stories about their super healing powers, but (pay attention!) the stories are bullflop. Their superpowers were dreamed up by marketing departments trying to sell products, not discovered by independent researchers. Slow Learners, please fill in the blank: when you buy expensive superfoods, you are paying a ridiculous amount of money for _____. (Hint: it comes from a cow's husband.) Good job!

3.   <u>Fruits and Vegetables – Eat Five Servings Every Day:</u> This is a classic example of a 'One size fits none' rule. The nutritional needs of a sedentary grandmother and her grandson the Sherpa are not the same. Here's a better rule: try to eat three portions of fruits and vegetables, plus one more for every 50 pounds or 25 kg that you weigh. Do you still want to get your fruits and vegetables from a magic pill you bought online, or from a green supplement that smells like seaweed, but with too much sea and too little weed? Y*O*U – A*R*E – A – S*L*O*W –L*E*A*R*N*E*R.

4.   <u>Kefir:</u> Kefir is a wonderful, healthy product that originated in <u>The Caucasus Mountains</u> centuries ago. Made from milk, it has properties similar to yogurt, and even tastes similar. Like yogurt, it has a variety of probiotic cultures that may be healthy for the digestive tract, and there is nothing wrong with drinking it – at least, there wasn't, until American manufacturers dumbed it down. The fat-free, sugary drink thickened with laboratory gums and brightened with artificial colors would be unrecognizable to the Eastern European cultures that originally developed kefir. Look for a natural, unsweetened version and add some fresh fruit.

5.   <u>Cold Cereal Is a Great Way to Start Your Day:</u> Every time I see children eating breakfast cereal from a box I cringe. Despite all the advertising from General Mills and Kellogg's, most <u>cold cereal</u> is miserable food. It will not help anyone, of any age. Why? Most cereals have three main ingredients: sugar, highly processed grains, and unpronounceable chemicals. The added sugar is usually high fructose corn syrup, which many experts say is very unhealthy and the rest say is extremely unhealthy. Before you eat cold cereal (or, G-d forbid, give it to your children), read the label.

6. <u>Wine Is Good for Grandpa's Heart:</u> Maybe, maybe not. A little alcohol may be good, but a lot is deadly. Researchers looked at the relationship between alcohol consumption and the heart in about 4,500 people whose average age was 76. The conclusions: older men should have at most two drinks per day; older women should have at most one. Otherwise, alcohol can do deadly damage to the heart's structure and to its ability to function. As I wrote earlier, Mormons do not drink, and they live seven years longer than the rest of us. And they smile all the time. Good advice.

7. <u>Coffee Prevents Erectile Dysfunction:</u> Wouldn't that be nice? This story raced giddily around the Internet, however, coffee won't replace Viagra any time soon (sorry, boys). This was a single study of 3,724 men who *self-reported* about caffeine intake, not about coffee (sorry, Starbucks). <u>The study's conclusions</u>: "Caffeine intake significantly reduced the odds of prevalent ED, especially an intake equivalent to approximately 2-3 daily cups of coffee (170-375 mg/day)." More than four cups and the benefit quickly deflated. Again, this was a single study of men who self-reported about how often they experienced ED. Men self-reporting about their own ED might be the only group in America that lies more often than Congress.

8. <u>Drink Gatorade When You Exercise:</u> Feeling dehydrated? Drink water, not Gatorade (and not fruit juice). The best thing I can say about a glass of Gatorade is that it is slightly less unhealthy than a glass of Coke. Gatorade is made from sugar, sodium, potassium – and water. Does anyone ever need it? Sure: athletes training on a hot field, people who exercise and perspire heavily for more than an hour, people who spend the day at the beach, and anyone else who has rapidly lost a lot of fluid. Otherwise, water is healthier than Gatorade, especially for children. Worried about potassium? Eat a banana.

9. <u>Coconut Water Is a Healthier Drink Than Gatorade:</u> Coconut Water has a better stealth marketing program than Gatorade, but it is valueless. S*l*o*w – L*e*a*r*n*e*r*s, please fill in the blank: when you buy expensive water, you are paying a ridiculous amount of money for _____. Good job!

10. <u>Alkaline Water Is Better Than Coconut Water:</u>   Your first question should be, "What the hell is alkaline water? Simple. It is a scam – the latest successful entrant into the "Some people can be fooled into buying anything" parade. The 'science' behind alkaline water is nonsense, and it has nothing to do with how human digestion actually works. Save your money. (Note to Slow Learners: give your coconut water to your monkey – he is too smart to drink alkaline water.)

I could continue, but the list of over-hyped superfoods is endless. Just remember this: no superfood can help a poor diet. Instead of searching for a miracle, aim for a "super diet" by eating a wide range of unprocessed, healthy foods every day.

Additional Reading:
<u>**Earmarks of Nutrition Quackery**</u>

<u>**Diet Trends That Drive Nutritionists Nuts**</u>

****

At the beginning of this chapter I used the term 'Fad Food Fears' to describe foods we avoid because everyone knows we should avoid them, and that after ten or twenty years almost no one avoids. MSG, gluten, olive oil, and other foods all fall into this category. If there is a meme to this chapter, it is that most of our food fears are based not on science but on flawed scientific studies and rumors.

All of that was the easy part of dieting. You can ignore what your friends tell you, read what serious materials you can and ignore the rest. The next chapter discusses difficult problems: how to deal with the overwhelming complexities of obesity.

Chapter 6: The Art of Dieting

Yes, Dieting is an art. It requires frequent attention and constant practice, or else you will lose your skills and start gaining. However, most people approach a diet with less effort and consideration than they would put into learning to use a Hula Hoop. Let's do better, by thinking about some of the finer skills required.

Remember this: your body, your habits, your brain chemistry, even your gut bacteria will fight you every day for years. That's why I strongly urged you to learn to maintain your weight before you start to diet. That initial preparation will make your new life easier to maintain – but not easy.

This chapter discusses some of the ordinary problems with your new lifestyle that will inevitably arise, and some strong solutions for solving them.

ﻌﻌﻌﻌﻌ

What to Do When Your Weight Loss Plateaus

Weight plateaus are miserable. We've all hit them; we all hate them. You diet successfully, losing a pound or two every week, and then suddenly, nothing. Your weight stays the same. Up a pound, down a pound, up and down again. Plateaus are the cause of countless failed diets and yet they are perfectly normal – the body loses weight at its own pace, and sometimes stores excess water weight for weeks or even months before releasing it.

Hitting a plateau is so common that an entire cottage industry has sprung up to cater to the problem. Google "weight set point" and you will get about 360K hits, mainly linking to sites trying to sell you a way to break through your plateau. (The methods may seem reasonable or magical, but remember this: none of it has been properly tested and the products don't work.)

One of the biggest reasons that people fail is that they don't know how to handle plateaus. They will diet successfully for a while and weight will drop off with some consistency, but then they will stabilize at a point well above their goal. Plateauing isn't the problem; the problem is that when they stop losing weight for a few weeks, they consider themselves a failure. And every dieter who thinks he or she is a failure will do the same thing: binge. I've done it, and chances are that you have, too.

The problem is that we set unrealistic goals for ourselves, fail to achieve the impossible, then beat ourselves up emotionally over the perceived failure. It took me years – no, decades – to understand this basic fact: when you hit a plateau, your body is learning how to stabilize at what will become your new, maximum weight. Again, your new, maximum weight.

A Plateau Can Be a Gift

If you look at it that way, a plateau is a wonderful gift. You may have to live at that weight for a few weeks or even months, as your body learns to accept its new norm, but be patient. Push too hard and your weight will bounce back up again. We dieters hate to be patient, but it is part of the process.

ଽ·ଽ·ଽ·ଽ·ଽ

What to Do When You Break Your Diet

How can you fix a broken diet? It's hard, but not impossible.

We've all been there. You start to diet, you lose some weight, and then you go to a party or to a vacation island or simply to the supermarket, and suddenly everything crashes around you. Weeks and months of carefully sticking to your program vanish as you break your diet with a sad splat, like a scoop of ice cream falling to the kitchen floor at midnight.

This happened to me recently, after more than thirteen proud years of control. I had two heart surgeries and my doc put me on three new meds. Meds that gave me gastritis. Heartburn.

Ulcer medicine isn't nearly as effective for gastritis as is ice cream, and within a few weeks I was eating the way I did twenty years ago, when I was morbidly obese. My stomach felt great, but the rest of me felt awful.

Fortunately, I had the tools to fix my broken diet. Regardless, the process was slow and brutal even though I write about wellness every week. I was successful and you can succeed too, with three surprisingly simple steps:

Three Steps to Fix a Stalled Diet:

1. Don't try to lose weight, just stop gaining.

2. Set reasonable, achievable goals

3. Follow The 16-Word Diet

Not what you expected, I'm sure. Regardless of whether you lost control yesterday or sometime late in the twentieth century, you want to start dieting again now. Today. This minute. You want to lose back the weight that you gained back as fast as you can.

If you reread that last sentence, you'll see how futile this approach is. Your goal is to lose back the weight you just gained back? What will happen if you 'succeed'? You'll gain back the weight you lost back after you gained... I can't type the rest.

No cycle was ever this vicious. However, if you follow those three simple rules, you can succeed.

You probably expected to see strong advice with severe rules: severely restrict carbs or severely restrict fat or severely restrict something ridiculous. Definitely something severe. That would be shallow advice, advice eternally repeated by dull-witted writers for dull-witted readers.

Here's the truth: the specific foods you should eat every day are the last thing to worry about. If you want to fix a broken diet, you must take control of your life first, so that you can control your eating. Let's look at these three steps again, because they should sound familiar.

Don't Try to Lose Weight, Just Stop Gaining

Stabilization is the first and most important principle of The 16-Word Diet Program. You can't successfully lose weight until you first learn how to not gain weight. It doesn't matter if you are slightly chunky or morbidly obese, you need to learn how to stop gaining before you do anything else.

Think of it this way: if you were driving in reverse but wanted to go forward, what is the first thing you would do? Shift into drive and gun the engine? Only if you wanted to crash. If you want to stop going backwards and start going forwards, the first thing to do is to... stop. Stop moving. Put yourself in neutral for a while until you are ready to move forward.

Losing weight requires the same discipline: to begin, you must stop gaining and put yourself in neutral for a while.

With the stress off, you'll be able to eat comfortably. Normally. Healthily. Once you can do that, you will have established a new top weight for your body. You'll know how to live happily at that weight, without ever going higher. You'll also have time to set smart goals for yourself.

Set Reasonable, Achievable Goals

A remarkable number of people select unachievable goals and then flagellate themselves when they fail. If you're intent on losing a massive amount of weight in a short time for some ultimately insignificant event, you'll quickly join the ranks of the Self-Flagellators. However, if you lose weight slowly, at a reasonable pace that never stresses your body, then instead of searching Amazon for a short whip you'll search for sunscreen that someone can rub on your newly attractive, unflagellated back.

This is the best way to diet successfully. It's slow, but it beats gaining all your weight back because you were too impatient. If you doubt this, remember what I wrote earlier: Dieting is like sex. Slower is better.

When you break your diet, this is all the advice you will need.

****

Falling off your diet is a common occurrence – we've all done it multiple times, and the simple suggestions above can jumpstart you. Here's another problem that's relatively easy to fix, once you recognize it.

৩৩৩৩৩

118

How to Avoid Bad Diet Advice

Bad diet advice is even more common than bad exercise advice. It lurks everywhere, waiting to confuse you. The worst comes from friends and relatives who, armed with iron-clad convictions, great enthusiasm, and deep ignorance, dispense glittery bull effluent.

Your friends and relatives will suddenly rave about the latest diet miracle touted by Dr. Oz, or the newest glittery herbal effluvium from Dr. Andrew Weil, or perhaps talk wisely about how to harness the slenderizing human energy field that surrounds you, as explained by Deepak Chopra. They will babble on, blissfully unaware that diet pills and diet herbal supplements do not work, and that energy fields only exist in science fiction.

A True Story

My friend Gretchen adores her German Shepherd, and so I was astonished when she told me that she had begun to give the dog raw ground beef, raw liver, and raw chicken.

Raw meat is a disaster – for dogs or people. It doesn't magically pop into existence in little white Styrofoam trays wrapped in Saran Wrap. It comes from some poor animal that was butchered in a slaughterhouse with utter disregard for sanitation, a place infested with every unholy species of bacteria to plague mankind since the first Caveman had diarrhea. Eating raw supermarket meat is like playing Russian Roulette.

I had to ask. "Gretchen! Don't you know how dangerous it is to give your dog raw meat?"

"My next-door neighbor says it's really good for them. She has been giving it to her dogs for weeks. She says they love it."

"Is your next-door neighbor a veterinarian?"

"No, she's a hairdresser."

Close enough. "Does she feed raw meat to her children?"

"No! That's disgusting! And they could get sick!"

Yes, they could. Especially when the dog sleeps with the kids. "Does she eat it herself?"

"Of course not."

"So why feed it to her dogs?"

"Because they like it!"

I decided not to mention the many things my dog would like to eat every time I take her on a walk. Instead, I changed the subject.

"Do you enjoy the meetings at Mensa?"

We Believe Our Friends, Not Our Doctors

We have all done what Gretchen is doing: we treat diet advice from our friends as if it is a Golden Truth. Studies have shown that, in general, people trust advice from their best friend more than they trust advice from their doctor. Ridiculous but true, because your friend is an idiot.

I decided to write this post after a friend told me that he had lost 65 pounds on the Blood Type Diet, and that I should try it. The basic concept is that the foods you should eat are determined by your blood type. There are four basic blood types, so there are four different 'ideal diets'. This is about as scientific as saying that since there are four basic eye colors, there are four different ideal shoe sizes.

BTW, I have no idea of how many basic eye colors there are – I just made it up. And you believed me, because we are friends. And I just said that your friend is an idiot. Wait a minute...

Bad Advice May Come from Good Sources

We are constantly barraged by bad diet ideas and bad diet products, hurled at us as if we were a wall – to see what will stick. Here are a few of the most obvious sources to avoid.

1. Never buy a diet pill, diet drink, diet tea, diet herbal extract, etc., that is advertised online or in a TV commercial. They are all bull effluent. No exceptions.

2. Never create your own diet unless you are properly trained. And no, reading Jane Brody every week does not qualify you as being properly trained.

3. Never take diet advice from your best friend, your mother, your neighbor, your partner, or your Aunt Sylvia whose idiot son Ralph lives

in her basement – unless your 'expert' has maintained a significant weight loss for a minimum of three years.

4. Never take diet advice from Dr. Emet Oz, Deepak Chopra, Dr. Andrew Weil, or any other charming snake oil salesman who promises that you will be cured of everything wrong with you if you just swallow a magic pill and put sunshine in your thoughts.

5. Never take diet advice from a personal trainer, chiropractor, naturopath, herbalist, homeopath, or even from a medical doctor unless he or she has had appropriate training. Obesity is a maddeningly complicated disease, not a sprained ankle. It requires a sophisticated, well-trained specialist, not an opportunistic MD or an herb-sniffing flower child who doesn't believe that the Seventies are over.

So – what should you do if you want competent help? Find an expert: a medical doctor who is an Internist or Bariatric Specialist, a Registered Dietitian (in Australia, an Accredited Practicing Dietitian), a nutritionist with an advanced degree, etc. Of course, experts are expensive. That's why I wrote this book.

Just be careful. If you consult with an expert who tries to give you diet pills or who puts every patient on the identical diet, your expert is a charlatan. Run away as fast as you can. Run as if your Congressman is walking towards you with his hand out. (If that doesn't frighten you, nothing will.)

A note to dog lovers and meat lovers: Yes, I know that many of you feed raw meat to your dogs and it hasn't hurt them. First, you may just be lucky. Second, I worry about contamination of supermarket meat; slaughter houses are open sewers. Third, I mourn the heartless way that gentle, domesticated animals were caged and then slaughtered. Fourth, I support meat that came from an animal brought down by a good hunter. It's healthier to us and more humane to the animal. Fifth, your dog's mouth (like most mammalian predators) is relatively germ-free. However, if your dog eats some supermarket meat contaminated with salmonella and a few minutes later licks your children, they might not fare so well.

જ°જ°જ°જ

Is There a Force-Feeder in Your Life?

We all have someone in our lives who tries to force us to eat. They are beautiful but dangerous Sirens, beckoning us to crash and join them on some exotic cluster of Greek islands full of ancient ruins. Thrilling, until you realize that the crumbling islands are really your Isles of Langerhans. (Sirens can be real bitches.)

Some of them try to guilt us into eating too much (it took me two hours to bake that pie!), some try to shame us into eating too much (you've lost a lot of weight – it isn't healthy! Slow down. Have more mashed potatoes.), or as a last resort, they dump food onto our plates when we aren't looking. They are force-feeders, trying to cram unwanted calories down our throats.

My wife and I were out to dinner with friends last month when an old friend, a woman we have known and loved since college, tried to sabotage my diet. It started as we approached the table.

"Jay! Wow! How much weight have you lost?"

Recently, I began to lose weight after a long plateau.

"Ten or fifteen pounds this year."

She congratulated me and then we moved on. I tried to order ahi tuna, vegetables and fruit. A normal restaurant meal.

"Have you ever tried sweet potato fries with your ahi tuna? Delicious! You can get fruit at home."

"Maybe next time."

Later. our friend insisted on ordering a giant dessert even though her husband had ordered a chocolate milkshake as an appetizer (I can't make this stuff up). She asked for four spoons and four dessert plates, then proceeded to give me a small portion I hadn't asked for.

"No, thanks – I'm trying to take off a few more pounds."

"Come on – we haven't seen you in months."

I didn't understand the connection between not seeing each other and my eating her dessert, but decided to be polite.

"Okay – thanks."

Five minutes later, she started to put more apple crumble and gelato onto my dessert plate.

"No more, please – it's delicious but I'm really full."

"No, no, no. Enjoy yourself. I can't finish this entire thing."

And she put more on my plate, which I ignored (almost). And then a few minutes later, while I was looking for the waiter (and an early escape), she dumped the remains of the now-soggy crumble onto my plate.

"Enjoy it! You've lost so much weight already! You look terrific!"

My old friend had turned into a force-feeder.

My Friend Wanted to Ruin My Diet

Apple crumble and vanilla gelato might not mess up my diet, but it could mess up my head. I looked straight at her, and wide, innocent eyes looked back at me. Too innocent. And then I understood. She *wanted* to mess up my head, to narrow the chasm that had grown between her husband and me.

In the 1980s and 1990s, her husband was athletic, handsome and desirable, and I was morbidly obese. But over the years the athlete turned into a couch jockey: his shoulders disappeared, his chest drooped, and he developed a watermelon-sized pot belly. I still have a grandpa belly, but I'm... normal-looking. My old friend no longer is, and his wife is jealous of the new comparison. That's why she wanted to force-feed her dessert to me. She wanted me to fail, to look more like my old self. And more like her husband.

The four of us will never have dinner again.

Learn to Spot the Force-Feeders in Your Life

Many of you have similar stories because often, the people closest to us try to undermine us. How often has someone urged you to eat a piece of cake, saying, "It's my birthday! Celebrate with me!" I've heard that whiny plea so often that I've developed a stock answer. "Of course. And will you celebrate with me on my birthday? I want to try naked skydiving."

People would never consider offering a drink to an alcoholic, saying "It's my birthday! Drink with me!" However, they will mindlessly urge us to overeat (Relax! It's a party!) or to have a mega-dessert because they baked it.

The problem isn't declining an offer of unnecessary food; the problem is recognizing the trap behind the offer. If it comes from a stranger, perhaps a server in a restaurant, it's easy to say "No." However, if it comes from someone you trust and love, it won't be so easy. If Mom says, "Eat this. It's delicious," it may be almost impossible to say "No". If your closest friend says, "Want to meet me for coffee?" it would be difficult to turn down a pastry. My suggestion: think of all the teenage baristas who breathed on that pastry before one of them puts it on a plate for you.

Somewhere in the small circle of your close family and friends there is at least one person who wants to ruin your program. Their motivations are hard to understand and probably unconscious, but they exist. Parents want to maintain control over their adult children; friends don't want to be outshone by their peers, etc. It doesn't matter who it is. If you can recognize the saboteur trying to ruin your program, you can evade their traps.

****

Force-feeders with their siren songs are easy to spot, and not hard to escape if you muster a little backbone. Crash dieting is even easier to stop: don't start.

ও৯ও৯ও৯

Crash Dieting Part 1: They Don't Work

Hitting a plateau is hard to cope with, but manageable. However, going on a crash diet and then breaking it is like falling off a cliff – you scream and flap your arms and curse the Gods, but nothing can stop your fall. That's why it's called crash dieting, not smart dieting.

Two mistakes explain most crashes: first, people start with no preparation; and second, they try to lose as much as they can, as fast as they can. Fatal mistakes. Quick weight loss is inevitably followed by quicker weight gain.

Here are stories about real people who failed. The first is about a man I know very well, and the second is about a group of people many of you knew well – or thought you did. Their stories seem unrelated; however, at the end of the day they are the same.

Bear and the Floating Honeytrap

Paul and I have been friends since the fourth grade. In the fifth grade, someone heard his mother call him 'Honeybear', and everyone has called him 'Bear' ever since. He is like family to me, even though he's a bit like the crazy cousin you love too much to put in a home.

Bear has always screwed things up in a remarkably public way, and he fell off his diet with all the grace and wisdom of Wile E. Coyote. Diet flameouts are always painful; his was a blowtorch. He started with the ridiculous theory that he wouldn't break his new diet if breaking it would humiliate him publicly, so he bet a reluctant friend that he could lose 100 pounds in a year. The stakes: the loser would wash the winner's car every weekend for 52 weeks. After making the bet, he sent an email announcing it to everyone he knew: friends, family, and colleagues. What could go wrong with that?

My friend Bear was always an idiot. Now, he is an idiot who is getting better at washing cars.

Bear's mistakes were pretty common. His diet was impossibly rigid, he lost too much weight too fast, and he didn't know how to recover once he went off his inflexible food plan. His slip was inevitable, even though slips can be controlled with the very first lesson of this book: learn to maintain your weight before you start to diet. Why? Because sooner or later, you are 100% guaranteed to eat something delicious but forbidden. You need to learn how to deal with it before it happens, not after.

We All Have a Little Bear in Us

Like Bear, most dieters fail in a predictable pattern:

1. They read about the latest *lose-weight-at-light-speed* diet craze.

2. They start the new program, adhere tightly to the new rules, and the pounds melt off.

3. They break their program in some completely forgivable way.

4. They feel guilty, begin to overeat again, can't stop, and the weight piles back on.

Sound familiar? I would call it the American Way of Dieting except that it started back when the first fat monkey came down from a tree and saw his belly reflected in a lake.

Most people think that their problem begins at Step 4, when they overeat. No. Their problem begins at Step 1, when they select a diet with all the care and forethought that they put into selecting lawn fertilizer. Then, at Step 2, they start their latest fad diet without preparing themselves properly. And so they fail, repeatedly. Anyone who thinks he can binge all day on Sunday and then wake up on Monday and 'be good' for the rest of his life is probably related to my idiot friend Bear.

Unfortunately, he didn't take that advice — or any other. He simply started a rigid diet *and never thought about what he would do when he stopped.*

Few of us think about what to do when we stop dieting, but that's when the hard part begins. Losing weight is difficult; maintaining a weight loss is hand-to-hand, mixed martial arts combat. If you don't train for it, you will be beaten to a pulp.

Bear Takes a Vacation

After seven months and 60 pounds, Bear needed a week off. He found a cruise ship with an excellent exercise facility and booked it immediately, ignoring the fact that, on a deluxe ship, gourmet food and mega-desserts are available 24 hours a day. It was like putting Bear in the woods and expecting him not to... slip.

Bear hadn't had anything sweeter than a cantaloupe for six months, and suddenly he was surrounded by tip-obsessed waiters eager to bring him giant ice cream sundaes and creamy lemon meringue pie and towering plates of chocolate cake and gleaming trays of chocolate butterscotch candies and everything else he had been dreaming of for all those hungry months. He would have had a better chance of holding out if they waterboarded him.

He cracked open like one of those cantaloupes he had been living on. Ultimately, he gained 77 pounds before he stabilized. It was the most he had ever weighed, even though he worked hard every weekend, washing a car owned by the reluctant friend who had warned him he would lose the bet.

Don't be a Bear. Plan ahead. Decide what you will do the next time you slip off your diet, whether it's for an hour or for a month. If you don't, you may end up feeling guilty enough to wash my car. Bear only has thirty weekends to go.

****

Most dieters make the same mistakes that Bear made. They start with no preparation and then try to lose as much as they can, as fast as they can, while exercising as hard as they can. Fatal errors. The faster you lose it, the faster you'll gain it back.

That said, Bear would have been even worse off if he had joined a weight loss center. You've seen them; they enable desperate people to shed tonnage at an unrealistic pace. Enabling centers are everywhere. They have a near-zero long-term success rate, but people eagerly throw their money at slender, charming closers while they fantasize over meaningless promises and dreams.

Let's look at a group of people who went into a famous program run by professionals, did their best, lost an astonishing amount of weight, and ruined their lives.

৯৯৯৯৯

Crash Dieting Part 2: They Can't Work

You have probably heard of *The Biggest Loser*, an obscene, life-wrecking reality show. It has a surprising secret: *The Biggest Loser* contestants, despite having the best (okay, the most photogenic) trainers and nutritionists that reality-TV-show money can buy, gained their weight back. Most of it or all of it, and sometimes more.

Why? Because the contestants were forced into a drastic diet and exercise regimen that focused on short-term results, not permanent improvements.

I've never watched *The Biggest Loser* (Hey! I have standards!) but its premise is well known. They find eight or ten people who are relatively young, reasonably healthy, and morbidly obese, then they put them on diets. The goal: to see who can lose the most weight during a single television season.

Contestants are herded together like cattle being prepared for slaughter. However, instead of being sent to over-crowded feeding pens to fatten up, they are sent to equally afflicted pens to slim down under the supervision of trainers wielding metaphoric cattle prods. Contestants are placed on semi-starvation diets and 'encouraged' to exercise for 8-10 hours a day, every day, for seven months. Also, while no one is looking, they may surreptitiously be given a variety of illegal diet pills. Cowboys never respect their cattle.

The herds have similar outcomes. Cattle gain massive amounts of weight while forced into weeks of unnatural, unpleasant inactivity, and contestants lose massive amounts of weight while forced into months of unnatural, unpleasant hyperactivity. In the end, the cattle are slaughtered by butchers wielding sharp knives and the people are slaughtered by reality, with knives sharper than any butcher's tools.

Boy, that was grim. But fun to write.

Scientists Study the Biggest Losers

Kevin Hall, an expert on metabolism at the <u>National Institute of Diabetes and Digestive and Kidney Diseases</u> who admits to a weakness for reality TV, had the idea to follow the contestants for six years to track their long-term progress.

He assembled a team that conducted a comprehensive, six-year study of the Biggest Losers; the research was funded by the NIH and published in the journal *Obesity*. The project was the first to measure what happens to people over long periods of time (up to six years) after they had lost large amounts of weight with intensive dieting and exercise. The results were astonishing: they showed just how hard our bodies fight back against weight loss.

For decades, researchers had known that almost every dieter, regardless of whether or not they are obese when they start, will have a slower metabolism when they stop. So they were not surprised to see that the Biggest Losers had slow metabolisms when the show ended.

The Conclusion: Their Metabolisms Were Ruined

What shocked the team was this: as the years went by and weight returned, the contestants' metabolisms did not recover. Nearly all the contestants have significantly slower metabolisms today than they did six years ago. Despite heroic exercise patterns (9-15 hours *every week*), they now burn significantly fewer calories than expected while at rest. Many contestants find that the pounds are continuing to pile on, as if their bodies were intensifying their efforts to pull them back to their original weight.

For example, Sean Algaier, 36, a pastor who lost 155 lbs. (70.5 kg) and then gained back 159 (72 kg), is burning 458 fewer calories a day than would be expected for a man his size and level of physical activity. Rudy Pauls, the electrical engineer from Massachusetts, now burns 516 fewer calories per day than expected. Danny Cahill, the musician from Oklahoma, now burns 800 daily calories less than is predicted – which is roughly as much as Kate Moss eats in, say, June. To stay in anything close to a 'normal' weight, these poor people must stay in a perpetual state of near-starvation, while exercising vigorously for the rest of their lives. That's physiologically and psychologically impossible. And a pain in the ass.

Dina Mercado, maintenance worker for Commerce, California, weighed 248 before starting. She dieted down to 174 and now weighs 206 pounds. (From 113 kg down to 79 kg, then up to 93.5.) However, she now burns 438 fewer calories per day than would be expected for a woman her size. (Note: this is her resting rate – before exercise. It is not possible for her to burn an additional 438 calories through exercise.)

Not every winner had disappointing rebounds. For example, Amanda Arlauskas, 26, a wellness coach and social media consultant in Raleigh, NC, went from 250 lbs. down to 163, then stabilized at 176. (From 113.5 kg down to 74, then stabilized at 80.) However, like Dina Mercado, her metabolism crashed. She now burns 591.1 fewer calories per day than would be expected.

The conclusion of the study: The Biggest Loser's intensive program actually made it harder for people to maintain a permanent weight loss. Very sad.

Set-Point Theory

Researchers have known about this phenomenon for decades. Called set-point theory, it was first defined in a National Institutes of Health paper published in December, 1990. (Set-point theory was understood far earlier, but scientists always believed it was a relatively short-term, fairly minor event.) However, no researcher expected that rapid weight loss would lead to a permanent, massive slow-down of the metabolism. Neuroscientist Sandra Aamodt wrote about 'The Biggest Loser' study in *The New York Times*:

"The root of the problem is not willpower but neuroscience. Metabolic suppression is one of several powerful tools that the brain uses to keep the body within a certain weight range, called the set point. The range, which varies from person to person, is determined by genes and life experience. When dieters' weight drops below it, they not only burn fewer calories but also produce more hunger-inducing hormones and find eating more rewarding.

"The brain's weight-regulation system considers your set point to be the correct weight for you, whether or not your doctor agrees. If someone starts at (a healthy) 120 pounds and crash-diets down to 80, her brain rightfully declares a starvation state of emergency, and uses every method available to get that weight back up to normal. The same thing happens to someone who starts at 300 pounds and crashed down to 200, as the 'Biggest Loser' participants discovered."

This coordinated brain response is a major reason that dieters find weight loss so hard to achieve and maintain. For example, men with severe obesity have only one chance in 1,290 of reaching the normal weight range within a year; severely obese women have one chance in 677. A vast majority of those who beat the odds are likely to end up gaining the weight back over the next five years. A report for members of the diet industry stated: "In 2002, 231 million Europeans attempted some form of diet. Of these only 1 percent will achieve permanent weight loss."

Sounds optimistic.

An Optimistic Note

Despite this gloomy story, there is hope for most of us. The Biggest Losers failed in part because their programs were so drastic. Also, their bodies didn't have sufficient resilience to bounce back from the trauma. Fortunately, few of us have gone on such a severe program for any length of time (forget about poor Bear). Better, many people have naturally resilient metabolisms that do not suffer long-term after a dramatic weight loss. I've lost 50-75 pounds at least five times, and my metabolism remains normal; you might have the same genetic good fortune. But don't push it.

Regardless, the solution to the problem of recovering from a crash-diet/rapid-rebound is clear: stop trying to lose weight; just try to stabilize. Eat healthy foods, follow The 16-Word Diet, and stabilize. Stay at your present weight for months, not weeks, while your metabolism heals itself as much as possible. Then, try to lose very slowly – two or three pounds per month, no more. Most likely, your metabolism won't interfere.

****

The most common way for crash diets to fail is on a holiday of some sort. Not holidays like July 4 when we have a single, joyous meal sandwiched in between normal living; crash diets fail on holidays like

Christmas or Easter, or vacations – occasions when we overeat for days or weeks.

જીજીજીજીજી

Christmas Holidays and Summer Vacations

What do the Holiday Season and summer vacations have in common? They are the times of the year that we are most likely to overeat. Deliciously tempting treats are everywhere, and half of the time they are free, giving us an infinite number of chances to prove the obvious: we are all food whores.

In fact, have you ever wondered why Santa is so... large? It's because we are overwhelmed by food during the holidays and we need a fat superhero to save us. From ourselves. We celebrate most holidays with a single mega-meal, but we overeat almost non-stop from Thanksgiving to New Year's. By January, we all need giant red suits.

And vacations aren't much better. We put on bathing suits and then eat as if it's Christmas.

Can you survive summer (or winter) vacations and the Holidays? Yes, without needing new clothes. The magic solution: eat like an adult. Don't binge and don't diet. Eat responsibly and you will be fine.

Some people may think this advice is superficial, but that means they missed the 'don't diet' part. Not dieting and not overeating *at the same time* is hard. However, maintenance is the only way to keep lost weight from finding its way back home.

Earlier in this book I wrote that people must learn how to maintain their weight before they can successfully lose weight; otherwise, sooner or later, they will break their diets and not know how to stop themselves. And then they will eat until they glow like Rudolph. The good news is that you can do better; it's the perfect time of the year to learn to stabilize your weight. If you can wake up in January and weigh what you weighed in November, you will have defeated Christmas Holiday Syndrome, which will put you into an elite group of winners.

Here's How to Beat the Holidays:

Five Basic Rules:

1. Resolve to keep your weight stable until January. It won't be hard; just eat like an adult, not like a kid who was recently adopted by Willie Wonka.

2. Start to diet on the first full day in January that you go back to work. I'm serious. Parties don't stop on January 1, so if you try to diet any sooner you might not get very far. Be patient.

3. Make a few long-term goals, but keep them reasonable. If you swear you will never swallow a gram of carbohydrates until you lose 100 pounds (45.4 kg), you will fail in a hurry. If you are 101 pounds overweight and your goal is to lose 100 pounds in a year, you will fail slowly. Again, be patient with yourself.

4. Weigh yourself tomorrow morning, before breakfast. Weigh yourself naked (cover the mirrors, you coward). That will establish your maximum weight from today until you start to diet. It may be a fat maximum, but who cares? The minute you focus on not gaining weight instead of on losing weight, life will get better.

5. Don't stop exercising, regardless of how much you overeat. If you do not exercise, don't wait for January. Ignore the weather and start today.

Five Specific Rules:

6. When you get to a party or other event; summon your inner camel. Drink a cold bottle of water as soon as you get there. It will fill you up and dull your hunger. Even more important, it will give you time to gain control of the situation.

7. Decide what you will eat and what you will not eat. For example, I never eat cookies, cakes, or pastries unless they are homemade. Good homemade baking always tastes better to me than store-bought, and if it isn't good I throw it away when no one is looking. This simple rule eliminates most of the desserts

that tempt me at any party. Create your own set of rules for eating at parties and follow them. Almost all the time.

8. **Food buffets are the enemy and the enemy is everywhere.** Look at every dish on the buffet, plan what you will take before you take anything, and stick with your plan. If you don't plan properly, you will eat like my friend Bear.

9. **Have very little alcohol.** It contains an enormous number of unnecessary calories, and worse, it will weaken your resolve. Stay strong.

10. **No marijuana.** You have a weight problem — do you really want to smoke a joint while surrounded by Christmas cookies, chocolates, and eggnog-flavored everything? If I smoked enough marijuana, I'd eat eggnog-flavored pork chops. And I stopped eating pork in 1974.

And with #10, we end on a high note. If you don't let yourself revert to high school behavior, and if you don't pretend that you can diet when the world is telling you to relax, you will be fine.

✱✱✱✱✱✱✱✱✱✱✱✱✱✱✱✱✱✱

Plateaus, breaking your diet, crash dieting, and overeating while on holiday are all common problems. Hard, but they can be fixed with a little common sense. That said, binge eating is far more difficult. The above fixes require plaster and a trowel; this next fix requires an artist's delicate hand.

৶৶৶৶৶

How to Stop Binge Eating

Binge eating is a difficult, emotional problem. It's heartbreaking. Bingeing is very different from the other problems in this chapter; those behaviors are miserable problems, but compared with bingeing they are relatively simple to control.

Binge eating is self-flagellation with no hope of redemption. It's uncontrollably gorging on ten-thousand-calorie meals every weekend for months or years, and hating yourself during every bite. It's staying up late half the time so that no one can see you eat the hideous quantities of crap that you hid during the day. It's leaving your office and having lunch alone every day, so that no one can see how much you eat. It's ordering insane quantities of candy online, so that no clerk can see you when you pay for it.

Bingeing is out-of-control, obsessive eating, as addictive as any narcotic. It can last for weeks or for years, and you don't know how to stop.

The most important thing to understand about binge eating is this: you *can* stop it. Not immediately – it would be ludicrous to pretend that a few words of advice can halt your binge and keep you from ever doing it again. However, you can learn how to turn future out-of-control overeating into mini-binges, and then into micro-binges, and happily live that way forever.

The Difference Between Overeating and Bingeing

Most people overeat occasionally, but it simply isn't an important element of their lives. We overeaters are different. Many of us binge two or three times a week, eating 5,000 or 10,000 calories at once, usually in secret.

When I was a lonely teenager, I would steal my father's car keys at least once a week and sneak out after midnight. I'd drive to the local White Castle, buy ten hamburgers, five orders of fries, and two chocolate milk shakes, and then eat everything during the short drive home. Did I hate myself? Of course. Could I stop myself? Not a chance.

Like alcoholism, binge eating is an addiction. It's estimated that at any given time, about 3.5% of women and 2% of men in the United States suffer from the disorder. Several times that many may have binged at some point in their lives; it's dismayingly common. Breaking the habit is brutally difficult, in part because the world is full of holier-than-thou snots who relish saying, "It's not hard. All you have to do is stop eating!!" How... empathetic of them. Especially the smokers.

The Basic Causes

There are two basic reasons for bingeing – biological and emotional. The biological causes should be healed first, while you work on the emotional issues.

Here are a few of the causes:

1. Gut Bacteria: As discussed earlier, each of us has a unique mix of different species of gut bacteria; in total, about 100 trillion bugs live contentedly in our intestines. Not surprisingly, long-term vegetarians and people on paleo diets have very different populations: vegetarians have a preponderance of organisms that live on plant-based materials, and paleo people have an abundance of bugs that like semi-digested meat. (That image is not the reason I stopped eating meat, but it keeps me in line.)

Someone who regularly binges on junk food will alter his gut bacteria: he will starve the healthy ones and cultivate vast colonies that love sugar and fat. And then, when those little beasties don't get enough sugar or fat, they will send chemical messengers to the brain demanding, "Feed me!" It's like Audrey in the Little Shop of Horrors, except it's you. As you cut back on binge eating, most of the unhealthy colonies die off. It becomes easier to eat normal portions.

2. Endorphins: Bingeing on junk food can have the same effect on the brain as bingeing on drugs, alcohol, gambling, etc. These behaviors cause the brain to release dopamine, serotonin, and other powerful endorphins that have a narcotic effect. Yes — bingeing, like heroin, gets us high. People tend to binge in the same ritualistic, secret pattern that alcoholic and other addicts often use: they buy the same high-calorie foods from the same out-of-the-way stores, eat alone in the same place, and then secretly dispose of the evidence. The entire sad, self-destructive pattern can repeat for years, even decades.

3. Psychological Reasons: People overeat for as many psychological reasons as there are unhealthy bacteria in Chris Christie's intestines. I can't list them all, but we instinctively know many of them. One important point: if you have read that binge eating is a 'bad habit' that can be broken or a 'learned behavior that can be unlearned', forget it. That is nonsense — pop psychology at its most foolish. Bingeing is a serious disease, and should be taken seriously.

A Typical Binge-Eater

My friend Cookie is an excellent example of a person who binges for complex emotional reasons. Cookie and I have been close friends since college, and I've never seen her overeat. When the four of us go out for dinner she orders the lowest-calorie, lowest-fat item on the menu. Green salad with no dressing. Broiled fish. Fresh fruit salad with cottage cheese, if she is feeling decadent. No explanation is necessary; Cookie is on a diet. In fact, she's been dieting for as long as I know her. And one last detail: Cookie is 5'3" tall and weighs 272 pounds (short cm, fat kg).

Cookie's diet doesn't work.

You already know why Cookie's diet is a giant belly-flop: her behavior is perfect in public but out of control when she is alone. Here's a question: when she is with her friends and eating so abstemiously, who does she think she is fooling? Not me. Not even you, and you've never met her.

I think we all have a little Cookie in us. When spending time with our friends or relatives, we want to prove we are in control of our bodies so we pretend to be perfect. "Get that crouton off my plate! It's a carb and it's ugly!" And then, when we get home and no one is looking, we break out a hidden bar of chocolate.

I Was a Binge-Eater for Decades

I binged for more than twenty years. I lived on hamster-portions during the day – when people were watching. However, once or twice each week I would sneak a half gallon of ice cream into the garage freezer, wait for my wife to fall asleep, tip-toe out, and consume – no, *inhale!* – the entire container. I lived that way year in, year out, until one afternoon, while watching a woman twice the size of Cookie eat three grapes and pronounce herself too full for lunch (you can't make this stuff up!), I had an epiphany: overweight people do it backwards. They diet in front of their friends and gorge themselves in private.

Simple Solution to a Complex Problem

I decided to turn my backwards eating pattern around: I'd eat whatever I wanted while out with friends but eat carefully when home, especially while alone.

The idea was both brilliant and ridiculous. (Hey! I didn't say the idea was modest!) I liked the honesty of it. My friends weren't idiots – I was over 320 pounds (145 kg) when I had this idea, and eating a salad for lunch wasn't fooling anyone, so why not stop pretending?

This simple idea was one of three changes that helped me gradually corral my binges while I shakily began to descend from that quivering peak. I switched from low-fat, low-quality foods to a protein-centered, high-quality program. I began to exercise, and when I was with my friends on the weekends I ate as if I weren't dieting.

It worked. By allowing myself to eat normally in public, I gradually became able to control my bingeing at night, at home, while everyone was sleeping. I didn't become perfect; I simply became closer to normal.

Often, I refer to this program as Dieting for Adults – a phrase that implies rigorous honesty. If you lie about what you're eating to your friends and family, then sooner or later you will compensate by bingeing at home, or in your car, or in some other safe, dark, private place. That's not Dieting for Adults, that's Dieting for Neurotic Teen-Agers.

It isn't easy to live a healthy life. The first step, learning the basics of a protein-centered diet, is child's play. However, adopting a healthy lifestyle and sticking with it forever, with few lapses, is harder than becoming a Navy Seal. Being honest with your friends and family about your eating is somewhere between the two: very difficult, but worth it.

How You Can Control Your Binge Eating

The cure for most binge eaters doesn't require pills or professional treatment. Instead, upgrade your microbiota with lifestyle changes: healthy foods and regular exercise. And with patience: the process is slow. Here are the simple rules:

- Follow the three rules of The 16-Word Diet.

- Find a friend or sponsor to talk with when you slip.

- Allow yourself to forgive yourself.

On a personal note (I have a lot of them), when I was in my late forties, Rule 2 kicked in. I learned to talk with my wife whenever I had a bingeing episode. She became the most powerful tool I had: an immediate brake I could apply whenever I started to slide downhill.

This is where most binge eaters (and dieters) fail. They try to succeed on their own, without finding someone to talk with, which is almost impossible. Addictive behavior can rarely be broken without help.

Finding a trusted friend is hard to do. A spouse or partner is not always ideal, and members of the clergy may not be available when you need them. Organizations such as Overeaters Anonymous may be a better choice; choose a sponsor who has had significant, long-term success with an addiction. Otherwise, your food sponsor could become your binge-eating buddy. Several online programs can help; try www.sparkpeople.com.

Finally, learn to forgive yourself. You wouldn't blame yourself if you caught the flu; don't blame yourself for having an unhealthy assortment of gut bacteria and an unlucky assortment of genes and life experiences. Instead, use the steps above, be patient, and you will do better. Also, regular, vigorous exercise will produce the same endorphins that junk food binges stimulate. Take it from someone who has binged countless times, few things are better than replacing a junk food high with an exercise high.

****

Now that we've talked about some of the things you should do, let's talk about some of the things you shouldn't do – whether or not it is holiday season.

Additional Reading:

The Science of Why We Binge

Binge Eating Disorder

****

And now, the saddest sentence in this entire book: when it comes to dieting, whether the topic is the complexities of bingeing or the basics of nutrition, every dieter is a s*l*o*w*-*l*e*a*r*n*e*r*. As I wrote in the introduction, we are all optimists, and we all hope for a magic obesity solution that doesn't involve a lifetime of careful living. That might happen someday, but not in our lifetimes.

One solution that really is almost magical is regular, vigorous exercise. It is the first line of defense against obesity, as well as the diseases of aging: heart disease, stroke, diabetes, even some forms of cancer. The next chapter explains why exercise is so vital to both your health and your figure; simply dieting isn't enough. The next chapter gives valuable guidelines and essential information.

Chapter 7: EXERCISE

Preface

There are things we love but do not need. We love Jay Leno and Dolly Parton, but we do not need to see them topless. And then there's chocolate. Love it, don't need it.

There are things we need but do not love. Oxygen and sweat come to mind. And then there's exercise. Need it, don't love it. In truth, it's a pain in the ass.

I love exercise as much as is possible for a man who has better things to do, such as taking a nap. Regardless, I exercise vigorously four to five days every week, because I plan to keep playing with my grandchildren until they have children of their own. And that is the heart of this chapter. People who exercise regularly live longer, healthier, more active lives than people who do not. If you are looking for magic in a bottle of pills, stop looking and start to exercise. It really is magic.

This chapter starts by explaining how exercise can and cannot improve your life. Yes, we give you a custom exercise program based on your WeightZone questionnaire; but frankly, anyone with Internet access can get far more exercise advice than I could possibly provide in one little book. What you cannot find – what is essential for your life – is how to summon the mental strength to begin a program after years or even decades of inactivity. If you do not get regular, vigorous exercise, then this is the most important chapter in the book. Please read it carefully and take its advice.

ഗ∞ഗ∞ഗ∞ഗ∞ഗ

Why Exercise Is as Important as Diet

Why is exercise so important if all you want to do is lose a few pounds? Because emotionally, your real goal is to look more attractive, and exercise is just as important for your looks as is weight loss. Sometimes exercise is more important.

I have a cousin who is like a sister. Three years ago she lost her husband unexpectedly; she mourned for a year before she was ready to re-enter the dating world. However, at 55, she was 90 pounds (41 kg) overweight and… disheveled. She needed to regain control. Her first move was to stop smoking: with so many single women past fifty competing for a few single men past sixty, she needed every edge she could get.

Next, she worked on her teeth – crooked and stained yellow from cigarettes and coffee. She found a cosmetic dentist who did an immense amount of work, put her in braces, and then six months later he did an immense amount of additional work. Fortunately, she could afford it, and ultimately her teeth looked wonderful.

After the braces went on, she had a gastric bypass – dieting had never interested her. Eventually, after losing more than 70 pounds, she had several rounds of cosmetic surgeries. First, her doctors removed the loose skin from her arms, legs, and belly, and then they performed liposuction to remove the fatty deposits that stubbornly refused to disappear from her calves and thighs.

However, she still lived in an aging body with an unhealthy lifestyle. She attacked that problem with her standard solution: she hired more surgeons. She had a face lift, butt lift, nose job, eye job, boob job, ear lobe reduction, and insisted that Botox be injected into every place that quivered.

When she was finally finished and had spent most of her husband's life insurance money, she looked, as the cruel old saying goes, "Beautiful from afar, but far from beautiful." She belonged in Madame Tussaud's, standing next to her surgery-soul mate Michael Jackson. She had transformed herself into an old wax mannequin with giant white teeth, only slightly more desirable than she was before she started.

Why Did All Her Cosmetic Surgery Fail?

My cousin did a spectacular job on restoring the outside of her body but ignored everything inside. Exercise? She never got off her couch, except to go to her next doctor's appointment. Healthy eating? Her diet remained – let's be gentle – self-indulgent, despite her gastric bypass, so her weight loss stalled. Essentially, if she could pay someone to make her look better while she was sedated, she would do it; but if the improvement required effort on her part, she wouldn't.

Today, despite joining every dating site in the English-speaking world, she is alone. She never gets asked out on a second date. One reason might be that she doesn't look healthy. Despite the glossy teeth and the wrinkle-free skin and the flat belly and the flab-free arms and the teen-aged earlobes and the perky boobs that she proudly shows to anyone brave enough to look, she remains... undesirable.

Because she refuses to exercise, the wonderful, shiny muscle tone she had as a young woman is gone. She moves like an old lady who hasn't gotten out of her chair for twenty years. Worse, she has the energy level of a blackout. Sometimes I want to shine a spotlight on her, to illuminate her, but she would suck out the brightness and remain in the dark.

The Best Way to Look More Desirable

The point is obvious. Regular, vigorous exercise and smart food choices – the basics of any sane program – will make you look robust and vital at any age. Sitting on your butt will make you look like a heap of melted marshmallows. Surgery can remove a few crusts, but so what? Without a healthy lifestyle, you will never look younger or more desirable. And isn't that the point?

I've given cosmetic surgery a great deal of thought since my cousin began her odyssey, and I've moved pretty far from where I started. I used to laugh at it, but I've grown compassionate. If optional plastic surgery is one part of a lifestyle change that helps someone improve his or her self-image, I'm all for it.

That said, I have a problem with older people who use cosmetic surgery as a substitute for a healthy lifestyle. The same people who once tried to look old enough to buy beer are now trying to look young enough to get laid. And in both cases, they can't fool anyone more sophisticated than a 7-11 clerk.

If a supposedly mature adult has a procedure to improve his or her looks but does nothing to improve his health, whom will he fool besides himself? What sane woman finds a sedentary grandfather with a sewn-to-the-scalp toupee and a Botox-injected forehead more attractive than a fit grandfather who is bald? What sane man finds a sedentary grandmother with a glazed face and store mannequin breasts more attractive than a fit grandmother with a few wrinkles?

Cosmetic surgery is fine as you age, but for goodness' sake, fix your insides, too. No 'age reversing' medical treatment is as sexy as is good health.

The following sections examine different areas of exercise. If you lead a sedentary life, please read them carefully. They were written for you. We'll start with a list of terrible excuses for not exercising – excuses we have all used.

৯৯৯৯৯৯

10 WTF Excuses for Not Exercising

The 10 Worst, Totally Foolish Excuses for Not Exercising will always be with us, used by friends and loved ones, because they are excuses, not reasons. If you want a healthier, sexier body but do not exercise, let's work on some of those Way Too Foolish rationalizations.

First, an observation. If you exercise regularly, even if you just walk your dog for 20 minutes a day, you are doing something wonderful for your body. If you like to read articles about exercise but you pay someone to walk your dog, then please turn off your monitor and go for a walk.

I'm serious. Go.

•••

I'd say "Welcome back," but none of you went anywhere. And that's the point: it is extremely difficult to motivate people to exercise once they have lived sedentary lives. And yet, exercise is the single most important thing you can do for your health. Yes, exercise, not a healthy diet. Why? Obviously, both are essential. However, people who exercise will naturally gravitate to healthy foods, but people who eat healthy foods do not naturally gravitate to exercise. Healthy eaters can be couch potatoes, but people who exercise cannot live on a junk food diet. Ask **Morgan Spurlock.**

Many People Are Full of... Excuses for Not Exercising

People who make excuses for not exercising are failing to observe The Rules of 'The Three Mosts':

>   1. Most of the time, eat healthy foods.

>   2. Most days, exercise.

>   3. Most of your life, stay happy.

Simple advice, but too many people hide behind elaborate justifications for why they cannot follow it. Here's a list of actual excuses I have been given by readers and friends. Let's look at why they are so transparently false and how to overcome them.

1. I don't have the time to exercise. Once you get diabetes and heart disease from lack of exercise, you will have plenty of time. For regrets.

2. It's too cold/it's too hot/it's raining. I remember that one – it's the old 'bad weather' excuse. I used it when I hadn't finished my homework. I was eight. How old are you?

3. I'm too old. No, you are not. If you are reasonably healthy, regular exercise will help you feel younger. And it will improve your sex life, or at least improve your memories of your sex life. Exercise will definitely stimulate something.

4. The air is polluted, so exercise does more harm than good. That's actually a reasonable excuse – until you drill down into the research. The short answer: if you are healthy but live in an air-polluted neighborhood, it is better to exercise than to remain sedentary. Regular exercise can increase your life expectancy even though it means inhaling dirty air. Masks that trap most particulate matter are easy to find online. They're a great way to release your inner super hero.

5. Every time I exercise my back/neck/knees/ankles/feet, it hurts.
    A. Find exercises that do not hurt your

back/neck/knees/ankles/feet.
   B. Find a doctor who can fix your
back/neck/knees/ankles/feet.
   C. Stop whining.

6. **I'm too tired at the end of the day.** If, say, you work in construction or wait on tables, you have a Get Out of Jail Free card. Just be sure to eat a healthy diet, avoid drugs (legal and illegal), and get eight hours of sleep. However, if your job is not physically demanding and you have fewer than five kids, please reread 5C.

7. **I can't start an exercise program. I'm out of shape!** What you are saying is, you can't do it because you haven't done it up until now. That may explain why you're still a virgin.

8. **I don't want anyone to watch me while I exercise.** That's a common feeling – I've been there myself. Two suggestions. First, you can go for a brisk walk every day and never see anyone you know. Second, you can exercise in your house. Treadmills and stationary bicycles are wonderful for cardio exercise. If you prefer, Google "indoor exercises". You'll find an astonishing variety of workouts, with and without equipment. If you are unsteady on your feet, Google "chair exercises" or "exercises for seniors".

9.   **My grandfather never exercised and he lived to be 87.**
Tell me about your grandfather.
    He was a mailman.
    Okay – so he walked every day?
    Yes.
    Did he smoke or drink?
    No.
    Go away.

10. **I don't need any excuses for not exercising! I don't like it and I won't do it!** Wow! Very impressive! You really sound like an adult!

Okay – you get the picture. The only legitimate excuse for not working out is a major health problem. Two valuable take-aways from this section: Remember The Three Mosts, and no more WTF excuses for not exercising.

ఴ౿ఴ౿ఴ౿ఴ౿ఴ

Does Exercise Slow Down Weight Loss?

"Exercise doesn't help weight loss. Marathon runners only burn 2,200 calories during a race, so a dieter would need to run almost two marathons to lose one pound." Did this pearl of wisdom come from Koko the Gorilla? No, it came from the director of a major weight loss clinic in San Diego.

Exercise confuses many diet experts. For example, Dr. Mehmet Oz has often disparaged the calories burned during exercise (sometimes, Dr. Oz sounds like Dr. Koko). Despite Oz and his 'expert' advice, exercise is the single best thing you can do for your body and for your looks. It may not speed the rate of weight loss, but it will help you lose fat and water while it gives you a trimmer, fit body. Much better than moving the needle on some scale.

Does Exercise Burn Many Calories?

Four simple facts:

1. The number of calories your body burns during a single workout is not important. What's important is the number of calories your body burns all day, every day.

2. When you lose a half pound (226 g) of fat, you also will lose about a half pound of water. That means that if you diet and exercise away one-half pound of fat, you will lose one full pound (0.45 kg). If you diet and exercise away five pounds of fat, you will lose ten pounds (4.5 kg) (approximately).

3. If you exercise regularly and vigorously, you will build muscles that burn more calories – all day, every day. Yes, even while you are sleeping. If your new muscles simply burn 25 additional calories per day, that's 750 calories per month, or

nearly a quarter pound (113 g) of fat. Add in the quarter pound of water that you lose, and those measly 25 calories mean you'll lose almost six pounds (2.7 kg) a year.

4. If you lose a pound of fat and water, and gain a pound of muscle, bone, and other healthy tissues, you will look and feel better. Your scale will not change, but so what?

Dieters Have Two Goals

We dieters have two primary goals: to get healthier and to look better. That means losing fat and adding muscle. If you diet and stay on the couch, you'll lose fat but you'll also lose muscle. However, regular exercise creates healthy, dense new tissues – muscles, bones, and more – while it targets your stored fat, so it will give you a sleek, firm look. By contrast, a pound of fat – so fluffy that it floats – takes up much more space on your body. Big, lumpy space. Dieters who exercise vigorously may slow their weight loss slightly, but they will be trading big and lumpy for sleek and firm. Much better.

And there is a bonus: active people stay sharper as they age – more mentally alert – because exercise strengthens the heart and the arteries, the feeding tubes for the brain. Ever see an ad for a program that claims it will 'exercise your brain' with puzzles and games? <u>No one is sure whether or not they work.</u> Worse, supplements that claim to "support healthy brain function" are a complete waste of money. "Supports healthy brain function" has no legal meaning. I could sell Tootsie Rolls with the claim that they support healthy brain function, and it would be almost impossible to stop me.

People who stay physically active as they age will retain their intellectual skills longer than people who don't. If you exercise your body and eat healthy foods most of the time, your brain will take care of itself – for free.

The Scale Is Not Your Friend

Health professionals and trainers who pretentiously say things like "A dieter would need to run almost two marathons to lose one pound," are encouraging us to focus on the scale, not on our bodies. They are amateurs. A pro would encourage us to work on making our bodies healthier and more attractive. That's the value of regular exercise: it diminishes the importance of the scale by making us stronger and sexier – at any age and at a broader zone of weight.

Here's an easy thought experiment: if by some miracle you could have a body like a swimsuit model and live an active, healthy, happy life until you were 120, would you care about how much you weighed? Of course not. You would never get on a scale again – your weight wouldn't matter. The only people who would care how much you weigh are the whores working for your insurance company; they would leap gleefully at a chance to raise your rates.

The problem is that too many people still believe the Kokos and the Dr. Ozes of the world. They worry more about their scale than they do about their exercise program. Are you one of them? Are you exercising regularly but feeling unhappy because you aren't losing weight fast enough? Okay – think about this: does Beyoncé care how much she weighs? I don't.

જી-જી-જી-જી-જી

Let WeightZone Help You Design Your Own Workout

Designing your own workout seems like a dopey idea – but it's not. Health club memberships cost hundreds of dollars per year, personal trainers cost several thousand, and most free sites offer cookie-cutter workouts to everyone. However, the WeightZone Fitness Analysis is free and customized to your body and goals. Spend a little time with it and you'll have a wonderful basic program for your needs, not for anyone else's. Still sound dopey?

Obviously, you can get much better guidance from professionals than you can get from any software applet, but not everyone can afford them. Also, many obese people prefer to exercise in private, without anyone looking at our bodies. (I was that way for most of my adult life, even though I grew up in a beach town and spent entire summers in a bathing suit.) The software I designed will give you a good, basic program based on the answers you gave to our questionnaire, and it will keep pushing you to do better as you get healthier.

You'll need a current WeightZone report; if you don't have one, go to www.weightzonefactor.com, take the test, go to your Results Page, and scroll down to the four big buttons: **Fitness Assessment, Target Heart Rate, Workout Schedule,** and **WeightZone Calculator**. Each button brings you to a new page with customized fitness advice based on your body stats, health history, and exercise history.

The WeightZone Fitness Assessment uses a popular tool called the Rockport Walking Fitness Test to estimate how fit you are for your age group. More important, it determines if your oxygen consumption is satisfactory. If you don't have a heart rate monitor, you'll just need a watch and the ability to take your pulse. (Remember to start counting from zero, not one.) If you get a high score on the Fitness Assessment, congratulations! If your score is low, check with your doctor.

The WeightZone Target Heart Rate tells you the optimum pulse to maintain while you exercise. Too fast is dangerous; too slow may not do you much good. The applet uses an algorithm I developed that gives you an optimal range in which to work out instead of an impossible-to-maintain magic number. However, here's a simple rule of thumb: If you exercise three to five times a week for thirty or more minutes a day, and if you work out hard enough to pant and sweat a little, you are getting regular, vigorous exercise. Again, check with your doctor.

The WeightZone Workout Schedule Is based on your present level of health and activity. It tells you how many days to do cardio exercise each week, how many days to do strength training, and how many minutes to work out each session. It also tells you how many sets and reps to perform. These recommendations are based on our proprietary mathematical analysis of your health and exercise history, and they will change as you continue to exercise regularly. Retest yourself every month or so.

The WeightZone Calculator is a powerful tool that shows how your WeightZone will change for the better as you improve your workouts. It also shows when you reach a point of diminishing returns; your numbers will stop improving. Enter different values for the number of days and minutes that you want to exercise, and the Calculator will predict your new WeightZone. It's a great way to motivate yourself.

Getting Started

WeightZone gives excellent, basic guidance to help you begin or improve a strength training program.

- If you don't exercise, it will start with a walking program.

- If you only do cardio, it will suggest a basic strength training routine, and give specifics about reps, sets, frequency, etc.

- If you already have a good program, our software will increase its intensity.

If you have not exercised for a long time, start slowly. Walk for twenty minutes every other day, then gradually go up to five days a week. Be sure to rest for a day or two each week, especially if you are past sixty. Slowly add five minutes per day until you reach 40 minutes, five days per week. You can add more time if you like, but the improvements will quickly diminish. When walking becomes easy, retake your WeightZone test to get an upgraded program.

If you already perform regular cardio exercise, add in strength training. Stop whining! Do you want to get old and ugly, or stay young and beautiful? If your response is that you are no longer young or beautiful, study the seniors who power-walk around a mall and then visit a nursing home. Which ones would you rather look like in forty years?

WeightZone does not suggest specific exercises (we hope to have a package ready soon). However, it's easy to find comprehensive workout routines online. At the end of this article, you'll find links to sites offering free strength training routines. Select your exercises based on the equipment and facilities available to you (if any), and your personal preferences.

Too Busy to Exercise?

Most people have the same excuse: "I have no time to exercise!" Yet somehow, they have time for their favorite TV programs. "Oh, I can't give up The Bachelorette! I have to know if Kaitlyn says yes to Shawn!" (No, I'm not exactly current with Bachelorette romances.)

Okay. Here's the hard part: how do you maintain an exercise program for years? Successful exercise programs are like successful diets: fun to dream about, easy to begin, and almost impossible to maintain.

I was lucky. After my first heart attack (that's not the lucky part) I entered cardio rehab and stayed for four months. I watched people come and go. Some whined from Day One. They didn't stay for long but they outlasted the over-enthusiastic loudmouths, who acted as if their goal was to become the first heart attack survivor to climb Mt. Everest and who quickly vanished into a snowbank somewhere.

The winners were the quiet ones whose driving goal was not to have a second event. They had faced their own mortality and, thoroughly humbled, had chosen to take charge of their lives. Those winners taught me how to stick with an exercise program: by focusing on an important, long-term goal, not a frivolous one.

If your goal is to look your best at a wedding/graduation/Bar Mitzvah/Communion/reunion/divorce paper signing/naked house party/ or something even weirder, then as soon as the event passes you will stop exercising, stop dieting, and your inner couch potato will blossom. If your goal is a long, healthy, pain-free life and if you never lose sight of that goal, you will succeed. Choose wisely.

****

Additional Reading:
The following sites give free strength training programs and advice. If you want more, Google "**Free Strength Training Routines**".

http://www.muscleandstrength.com/workouts/main.html

http://exercise.about.com/od/exerciseworkouts/u/workouts.htm

http://www.fitnessmagazine.com/workout/

୭୭୭୭୭

Five Easy Rules for Your New Exercise Program

Every type of exercise is valuable, as long as you follow some basic rules:

Work out regularly

Depending on your condition, 3-6 days each week is best, for 20-60 minutes. Don't start at full blast; start slowly, gently, and build up until you reach the limit of your comfort zone. Think that you don't have the time to work out? Nonsense. You can exercise in five-minute intervals: before you go to work, on your lunch hour, before dinner, etc. Or, if you just exercise for 20 minutes on Wednesday, Saturday, and Sunday, both your body and your health will improve.

Exercise your entire body, not just your legs

Start by performing strength training exercises to build your upper body. Perform core exercises to build your stomach and back. After a few months, the improvement to your appearance will be obvious. And the older you are, the more important it becomes to exercise your whole body.

Don't take it easy

One common rule is to exercise hard enough so that it is difficult to whistle while you walk. Another is to work out hard enough that you are mildly out of breath and sweating slightly. And don't take your friend's opinion unless she can show you her degree. Ask your doctor or certified trainer.

Don't get into a rut

Mix things up. Try to perform several different types of exercises each month. This way, you will use different muscles in different ways. You will gain endurance, look better and have fewer injuries.

Grow your endurance, not your muscles.

Most men (and some women) think that what's important is growing giant muscles that make your shirt bulge. That's okay, but not important. What's important is growing endurance. Better for your heart, better for your joints, essential for a long, strong life.

You are never too young to need regular, vigorous exercise; you are never too old to start. The next section explains Rule #5 nicely.

 و-و-و-و-و-و

How Strength Training Helps You Lose Weight and Look Better

What's the most effective way to improve your body? Strength training. Dieting helps you lose fat, but strength training will make you look and feel more vital.

Whether you're an old woman or a young man, if your goal is to lose weight and get a slimmer, healthier body, then strength training is the fastest, surest way. You can start today, without any equipment, and see the difference next week.

When they hear the term 'strength training', most people think of grotesque steroid freaks lifting insanely heavy barbells. No. Strength training simply means exercising the muscles of the upper and lower body so that as you age, your body will stay young.

In 1997, when I began strength training, I looked twenty years older than I was. Today, I look twenty years younger than I am (in my own inflated opinion). Strength training will do that for you: it will improve your looks and, more important, your self-image. I cannot overstate how much better my life is today: after decades of obesity, I finally fit into my own body. If you feel your stomach lurch away from you when you rise up from a chair, or if you sit down and feel your butt hit the chair before it should, then you understand. Somehow you have become trapped in a body that doesn't fit. Smart exercise will help you escape, regardless of your age.

Let's look at the benefits, and then at some simple ways to work strength training into your busy life.

Benefits of Strength Training:

1. Help keep weight off permanently.

2. Burn more calories 24 hours a day. (Yes, even while you sleep. All those new muscles will be generating heat.)

3. Prevent loss of bone density (osteoporosis) and loss of muscle mass (sarcopenia) as we age.

4. Reduce risk of Type 2 Diabetes, may lower insulin needs.

5. Improve balance, coordination, and posture. That is the difference between "feeling your age" and "feeling young".

6. Gain endurance for everyday tasks, get more energy during the day, and better sleep at night.

7. Increase HDL – High Density Lipoprotein (good cholesterol) and decrease LDL – Low Density Lipoprotein (bad cholesterol).

8. Lower high blood pressure and risk of cardiovascular disease.

9. Rehabilitate injuries and reduce chronic pain.

10. Get a better body for very little effort. (Send me pictures.)

And most important,

11. Improve your sex life. (Yes, seriously. If weight loss and regular exercise do not improve your sex drive and performance, visit your doctor. A low sex drive can be a symptom of a serious medical problem.)

Does Strength Training Fit into Your Lifestyle?

You may be thinking: "Nice list, but not for me." You are not into strength training or gyms, and definitely not into lifting weights on a sticky bench after strangers wearing sweaty shorts sat on it. Good for you. If you want to watch a group of people sweat and grunt while they ignore what everyone else in the room is saying, you can sit on a couch and watch cable news.

However, if strength training isn't for you, I have a question: Which of the above ten points are you specifically not interested in? Which benefit do you not want for your body?

If you are serious about weight loss, get serious about strength training.

If you can afford a gym membership or a home gym, and if you use it faithfully, you're my hero. But that's a big 'if'. Affording it may be hard, but using it faithfully for more than a few weeks is almost impossible. The best way is with a workout buddy who has a long, steady history of regular exercise.

Alternatives to the Gym

Like many people, I do not belong to a gym or own expensive equipment; I prefer to exercise outdoors in the fresh air and sunshine. How? I strength-train my upper body while walking my dog. It's fun, and all that simultaneous movement of arms and legs creates a great cardio workout. (It's easier than it sounds — you can use resistance cords, ultra-light weights, etc. Just don't trip and hurt yourself.)

There are many effective, inexpensive ways to strength-train while doing something that you enjoy. Calisthenics or body weight exercises such as push-ups and crunches are excellent. You can buy an exercise mat, put it in front of your bed, and exercise while you watch cat videos on YouTube. Resistance cords are wonderful and cost just a few dollars. They are especially good for seniors afraid of losing their balance; seniors can use resistance cords while sitting in a sturdy chair.

If you want to exercise your upper body while walking, start with the smallest possible weights: 1 or 2 pounds (0.5 kg - 1 kg). The goal is not to lift heavy weights; it is to move your arms in every possible direction. That means performing as many different exercises and as many repetitions as you can. Why? Because unless you are an insecure teenage boy you don't need massive muscles, you need flexibility and endurance. Something as simple as walking with your hands over your head (without weights) is a wonderful start; it's surprisingly effective cardio exercise and it can improve the strength and the range of motion in your shoulders.

A Quick Summary

Give yourself a few weeks to learn what works best for your body, and then every time you take a walk you'll get comprehensive upper-body exercise and an excellent cardio workout. The effect on your body (and your body fat) will be dramatic.

How often should you do strength training? Two to three times per week, for fifteen or twenty minutes per session, is a great start. As time goes by, you can add a few more minutes or make the exercises a bit harder. And remember: never stop, ever. If you take a week off, whether it's for a vacation or a heart ablation, target a realistic date to start exercising again and stick to it.

If you do strength training-exercises and eat fresh, healthy foods, then everything else will fall into place — permanently. And that is the secret of life.

Additional Reading:

Strength training Is the Best Way to Lose Weight

Strength training improves your sex life

Will exercise boost testosterone levels?

How to start a strength training program (SparkPeople.com)

Lifting weights can control blood sugar

ುುುುುುುু

How Much Exercise Is Enough?

According to several new wellness studies, people who exercise moderately live longer than people who exercise too much.

Surprise!

For decades, we have all worshipped The True Gospel of Exercise, absorbing endless sermons from the American Heart Association, The Mayo Clinic, and others: Exercise for a minimum of thirty minutes a day, every day, and more is better. Except...

Except for one problem: The American Heart Association and the Mayo Clinic are run by giant ferrets in white lab coats who waste so much time running on giant ferret-sized hamster wheels that it takes several decades for them to learn something new. And those white-coated ferrets have been too busy spinning their wheels to bother studying actual athletes, to see the actual effects of extreme exercise on the actual human body.

Good News (for Most of Us)

This should chase away that image of giant ferrets. Several groups of researchers have published results that should surprise no one: moderation beats extremism, in both dieting and exercise.

A meta-analysis in *The Journal of the American Medical Association* reviewed data from nearly one hundred large epidemiological studies, to determine the correlation between weight and mortality risk. The results: adults categorized as overweight or obese by their BMIs have a 5-6% lower mortality risk than "normal-weight" individuals. Lower, not higher. For example, given a group of women who are 5 ft. 4 in. (163 cm), the ones who weigh between 108 and 145 lbs. (49-65 kg) have a higher mortality risk than do those between 146 and 203 lbs. (66-92 kg) Chubby-but-healthy men have similar, surprising stats. (FYI, the BMI is an excellent tool for describing large groups of people. It just doesn't work for individuals.)

In our society, a flat, muscular abdomen and well-defined chest muscles are hallmarks of health and sexuality. Alas, they can also indicate a shorter lifespan. A six-pack is fine if you are in your twenties, but once you pass forty it's time to add a few pounds. Not a few dozen, but enough to protect yourself from the many illnesses that can burn through your body's resources like money in the hands of your congressman. (Assuming you don't own him, of course.)

Too Much Exercise May Be Harmful to Your Health

Isn't more exercise better? Yes, but only up to a point. We should all take a couple of days off each week. Muscles need time to rest, so that they can grow new tissue and repair the damage from previous workouts.

Two studies in the British journal *Heart* add new evidence that extreme exercise may be unhealthy. One study followed 1,038 patients with heart disease for 10 years, and found that those who exercised daily and vigorously were more than twice as likely to die of a heart attack or stroke as those who exercised only two to four days a week. (Not surprisingly, those who exercised rarely or never had the worst outcomes.)

The second study adds to the substantial evidence that too much endurance exercise increases the risk of atrial fibrillation. The category of "too much endurance exercise" excludes most of us, but those of you who run marathons might want to stop gasping for breath long enough to ask yourself this question: "Why the hell am I running marathons?" If your answer doesn't include an enormous amount of endorsement money, take a nap.

Of course, vigorous exercise is wonderful for your body — if you limit yourself to 2 to 5 hours a week. For example, epidemiological studies of walkers have found that brisk walkers tend to live longer than casual strollers do, even if they exert the same amount of energy.

Lead researcher Dr. Michael Conkright said, "The good news is that intensity is a completely relative concept. If you are out of shape, an intense workout could be a brisk walk around the block. For a seasoned runner, it would require more effort." In short, vigorous, heart-pounding exercise is dramatically better for the body than, say, pancake flipping.

Finally, just to confuse you a little, a study of the long-term results of exercise on marathoners, tri-athletes, etc., shows that their hearts end up just as healthy as people who exercise moderately. That's probably reassuring to the long-distance athletes in the world, but none of them are reading this book. More important, they spent more time running than most of us do eating, and their hearts don't end up any healthier than ours are.

Expert Advice Keeps Changing

And so, two more solidly held beliefs are turned upside down like a salt shaker (salt has changed from being a killer to being just another condiment). Now, we know that skinny long-distance runners with granite abs and gorilla glutes aren't nearly as healthy as they think they are.

What can we learn from this massive confusion, other than to follow the ancient Roman dictum 'Moderation in all things'? Read this carefully, because it is very important. Remember that obnoxious girl in high school who had a perfect body and who didn't gain a pound after she had three kids? The one who married the skinny, gorilla-gluted marathoner? Remember how they used to ignore you when they passed you in the hallway? You will probably outlive them both by ten years. As you should.

Additional Reading:

Too Much Exercise May Be Harmful to Your Health

Overweight Americans Have the Lowest Risk of Premature Death

<u>Hardest-Working Athletes Are Most Likely to Develop Atrial Fibrillation</u>

<u>Right and Left Ventricular Function and Mass in Male Elite Master Athletes</u>

****

Now, let's look at a different problem: an enduring exercise myth that is completely false but that will not go away. Which myth? The myth that claims you can tell your body where you want it to lose weight and it will obey. Your kids don't do what you want, so why should your hips?

෨෨෨෨෨

Will Spot Reducing Shrink Your Belly Fat?

Spot reducing. Everyone tries it; everyone fails. Why won't our bodies cooperate?

In a perfect world, we'd exercise a flabby body part a few times and watch the fat disappear. Crunches would shrink bellies, stationary bicycles would silence thunder-thighs, and we'd all have glorious, sculpted bodies. Unfortunately, the world isn't perfect. For dieters, it sucks.

Here's the truth: spot reducing doesn't work. Exercising your stomach muscles won't shrink the pad of fat over your tummy. Exercising your arms will not eliminate those bingo wings, and any pill, lotion, or diet that claims it can help you lose weight from specific areas of your body is a scam.

Some of you are thinking, "No, no. Crunches will definitely reduce my belly fat. My trainer told me they would, and his stomach muscles make my knees weak." Three questions:

- Does your trainer have excess fat anywhere on his body?
- Have you ever seen anyone who has well-defined abs but whose arm flab sways when she scratches the back of her neck?
- Is your trainer a member of <u>Mensa</u>?

No one has wonderful abs in isolation; they have wonderful bodies, with no excess fat anywhere.

Can Supplements or Exercise Help You Spot Reduce?

Magic pills and miraculous exercises cannot help you spot reduce; the entire concept is nonsense. Your body has hundreds of billions of fat cells, each with a microscopic drop of fat and a microscopic drop of water. When you lose weight, you burn fat and eliminate water, one cell at a time. How does your body choose the specific cells it uses? No one knows. And no one can control it. The person who solves that fundamental medical question will win a Nobel Prize. (Frankly, I think there should be a Nobel Prize for wellness writers who refuse to pimp worthless diet products, but the Committee hasn't called me yet. You should give them a hint.)

The process of weight loss is very complicated. Dieting is self-starvation (ouch!), and evolution has created many safety mechanisms to fight it. As one evolutionary result, the inches you lose will not be evenly distributed over your body; worse, the stomach is usually the last place to give up extra fat. (For some women, it is the hips.) And men, pay attention: as you age, your excess fat may drift to the pads over your stomach, even if you lose weight. It's as inevitable as back hair (an image you ladies did not need, but this is a science column. Sorta.).

After all the gloom, there's good news: spot exercises build muscles in the right places. As you lose weight, those muscles will pop. You might not look like a model in a magazine, but you will look very good. That's why you need 'smart goals': they aim for the best your body can achieve without being unrealistic. If you are a woman who has had two children and you want a slinky body with perfectly toned abs, don't look at pictures of Jessica Alba and say, "If she can do it, I can do it." She can afford an army of private nutritionists, personal chefs, and super trainers; you can't. And her pictures are professionally photoshopped – you are stuck with blurry selfies.

That said, if your goals are reasonable and you lead a healthy lifestyle, you will do better than many celebrities, long-term. Just think of Arnold Schwarzenegger. He was Mr. Universe four times, but these days, any decent grandpa bod is as good as the sad Arnold bod. My body is no worse than his, and I can assure you that there is not a single woman in the entire State of California whose knees would go weak if she saw me with my shirt off. All those steroids and cigars finally caught up with Arnold, just like Maria did.

The Best Way to Improve Problem Areas

Back to real people. Is there a way to lose flab that has accumulated in unpleasant places? Sure, but it isn't fast and it definitely isn't easy. Think long-term. Don't expect to build a perfect body in a few days or weeks; plan to keep improving for months and years. Remember that trainer with the impossibly perfect body? He wasn't fat and out of shape six weeks ago, or six months ago. It took him or her years of hard work. However, the hard work paid off for your trainer and it will pay off for you – if you adopt reasonable goals.

Reasonable goals, not miracles. And if you are ever again tempted to spend your money on a new spot reducing system, remember this story:

Occasionally, I'm approached by someone selling a spot-reducing program who promises he will make me rich – crazy rich!!! – if I endorse his secret formula or secret exercise program or secret *something* that targets a specific area of the body. My response is always the same: "Terrific! I'll offer it to my readers as soon as you show me clear evidence that it works. Show me real, scientific proof from an independent science laboratory, not a testimonial from 'Reporter Samantha Barston in Tacoma' that was really written by Murray the Hack in Brooklyn. Send me proof that your spot-reducing miracle actually works, and I'll recommend it to all of my readers."

I'm still waiting to get crazy rich.

৵৵৵৵৵

Exercise or Diet: Which Is More Important?

This chapter opened with a section explaining why exercise is as important as diet. Now, let's finish with a section explaining why, in the long run, exercise is often *more* important than diet. This topic is even more personal than the earlier one; I wrote it five days after having heart surgery. If you change just one thing in your life after reading this book, make it this: start an exercise program. It will improve your life.

Recently I had stents put in to unclog four arteries – I have terrible genes. My father had nine sisters and brothers, eighteen nephews, two nieces, my brother and me. One sister died long before he was born. The rest of us (all thirty!) have had one or more heart attacks. Most of us also had Type 2 Diabetes, and the ones who never developed diabetes died in their thirties and forties of heart disease (diabetes never had time to develop). With one exception, those who made it into their late sixties were wasted shells of their former selves; think of old men sunning themselves and waiting to die.

The one exception I mentioned is a cousin who is now 87. He has slowed down a bit but remains razor sharp. I'm in late middle age with five heart surgeries behind me, and yet I, too, remain strong. We have the same, miserable genes, so why have we beaten the odds? Why are we alive, and free of diabetes?

Regular, vigorous exercise.

To be fair, our older relatives didn't have the benefit of modern medical technology, which has saved us both. To remain fair, our older relatives led unhealthy lives: they smoked, drank, sat whenever they could, and rarely ate vegetables or fruit. My 87-year-old cousin now lives in Colorado, where he continues to ski and hike. He has led an exemplary life, free of unhealthy habits, and the results show. We share the same miserable set of genes, yet we have remained vital for decades longer than our relatives. Modern technology and research helped, but exercise kept our insulin mechanisms healthy enough so that Type 2 Diabetes never set in, and kept our cardiovascular systems healthy enough to withstand multiple surgeries. Even better, exercise kept our minds sharp enough to care.

The stenting procedure I had five days ago was my third in ten months. The four stents inserted during the first two surgeries had clogged up with new tissue growth and needed to be cleaned out. (Miserable genes.) The day after the most recent surgery, I read a provocative article by UK cardiologist Aseem Malhotra. Published in the *Washington Post* in May of 2015, it remains popular today. The surprisingly simple premise: exercise will not help people lose weight, only dieting will. Weight loss, not cardiac health, is apparently his top priority.

For a minute, I thought that ducks were flying over my hospital bed. I heard quacks.

A Weak Defense

To be fair, in his article he defends himself from that attack – but so weakly, in so few words, that it didn't matter. According to Dr. Malhotra, "The idea that our obesity epidemic is caused by sedentary lifestyles has spread widely over the past few decades, spurring a multibillion-dollar industry that pitches gadgets and gimmicks promising to walk, run and kickbox you to a slim figure. But those pitches are based on a myth. Physical activity has a multitude of health benefits – it reduces the risk of heart disease, Type 2 Diabetes, high blood pressure and possibly even cancer – but weight loss is not one of them." And then he goes on to talk about weight loss.

Malhotra is a cardiologist. Where the hell are his priorities? The day after I read that article I was home, walking over a mile a day, and back to researching and writing. Exercise saved my life, not mere weight loss. Weight loss definitely helped by reducing the burden on my heart, but regular, vigorous exercise for over twenty years gave me the strength and vitality I needed to walk significant distances two days after surgery. Also, here I am researching and typing instead of sleeping, as most cardiac patients do. Thin, sedentary patients my age could barely muster the strength to use the TV clicker.

After that lengthy, self-congratulatory prelude (I warned you it would be personal), let's look at studies that compare obesity levels, fitness levels, and long-term health outcomes.

The Obesity Paradox

A study by **The Cooper Institute**, a nonprofit organization in Dallas, looked at body composition and fitness levels in 22,000 men, ages 30-83. Over the course of the eight-year study, 428 participants died of cancer. Those who were overweight and fit were two times *less likely* to have died than those who were lean and fit. Also, there was no significant difference in the overall death rates between the overweight fit men and the lean fit men. Many recent studies have confirmed these findings (see links below.)

Despite the claims of the many Dr. Malhotras of the world, obesity is not an epidemic – not unless having a healthy body that society considers undesirable is a disease. If obesity isn't an epidemic, what is? Heart disease and Type 2 Diabetes, when caused by sedentary lifestyles or diets that get too many calories from processed foods and sugars.

An obese person can live a long, healthy life if he or she simply follows The 16-Word Diet: eat mainly healthy foods and exercise regularly. Obviously, this doesn't apply to someone who is morbidly obese, but a person can have a potbelly or a larger-than-stylish tush and still lead an active, productive, happy life that extends to the end of his or her natural limits. If that describes you, the only thing you need to reduce is your load of guilt.

Here's a simple thought experiment. Think of fifty-year-old identical twins. One is definitely obese, but he exercises regularly and has a healthy diet. The other is at a perfect weight, but he leads a sedentary lifestyle and lives on junk food and beer. Which brother is likely to live longer? More important, whose body would you rather live in? The active brother with the healthy lifestyle who happens to be overweight, or the dull slug who happens to be thin?

The Cult of Slender

A personal story (this section is loaded with them). My mother was once hospitalized with a major health issue. Bedridden for months, food nauseated her. Every time I told one of her friends that she couldn't eat, I would be interrupted with an optimistic smile. "Think of all the weight she is going to lose!" They weren't wrong: Mom was on her way to being very slender and very dead. After she recovered, she gained back much of the weight she had lost, and got healthier.

When it comes to obesity, we are incapable of rational thought. We have been brainwashed by the Cult of Slender – so convinced of its value that we have forgotten how unhealthy Slender can be. We know the two best reasons for losing weight – get healthier and to get sexier – but we forget which goal is more important.

Exercise Creates Natural Bypasses

Everyone knows that exercise is important, but few realize how important. If you have a coronary artery that is beginning to block up, then regular, vigorous exercise may cause the heart to grow new 'arteries', called 'collaterals', that bypass the blockage and supply fresh blood where it is needed. They may prevent a heart attack.

Collaterals start life as hair-thin capillaries, the smallest blood vessels in the body. They bring oxygen, water, and other nutrients to individual cells, and carry away waste products such as carbon dioxide. The heart muscle is fed by countless capillaries that are unnoticed until a coronary artery begins to clog with plaque. If it closes completely or if a piece of plaque breaks off and blocks the artery, then the blood-starved section of the heart will die. That's a heart attack.

However, when blood flow begins to decrease through a narrowing artery, one (or more) capillaries may grow until it becomes a new 'artery'. Ultimately it will bypass the blockage, delivering fresh nutrients to blood-starved tissues and avoiding a heart attack. But this miracle isn't random; it is the result of regular, vigorous exercise. It will not happen if your idea of exercise is watching Monday Night Football. A better idea: listen to the game on your smart phone while you walk for a few miles.

Once Again. Exercise or Diet – Which Is More Important?

And this brings us back to Dr. Aseem Malhotra, the cardiologist who wrote in the *Washington Post*: "Exercise – no matter how many gym memberships you buy or how often you wear your Fitbit – won't make you lose weight."

Losing weight will allow you to fit into smaller-sized clothing. Exercising will keep you alive and healthy. Dr. Malhotra should re-examine his core values. He has a close-up view of them with his head so far up his ass.

We don't have an epidemic of obesity; we have an epidemic of inactivity. Obesity isn't killing millions of us prematurely because of heart disease; lack of exercise and a diet of junk food are. (Links below.)

One last thing. Above, I described myself as being middle-aged. All the people in the hospital who cared for me described me as middle-aged, from the cardiac surgeon who expertly inserted my new stents to the poor nurse who had to shave me with an electric razor when she really needed hedge clippers. I'm middle-aged, even though I was born in 1945. I'm seventy. I'm writing this chapter a few days after heart surgery. An old man couldn't do that. I am a healthy, middle-aged, active, seventy-year-old man, with a grandpa's belly that I plan to have for the next thirty years.

Too many physicians refuse to understand what they see every day – people who are 'overweight' by societal standards but who are healthy and strong, and who have extended their life expectancies through smart choices. Doctors keep insisting that we must lose weight, but they are ignoring countless studies that say lifestyle, not some number on the bathroom scale, is the most important factor. People who exercise live longer than people who do not. It's time that the medical profession stopped treating a non-existent 'obesity epidemic' and started promoting healthy lives.

There's been a strong theme running throughout this chapter: people overemphasize the importance of weight loss and underestimate the importance of exercise. I'll repeat the easy guidelines: losing weight will make you a lot thinner and a little healthier. Exercising will make you a little thinner and a lot healthier. And sexier than a slightly thinner slug.

Your choice.

If you have a good exercise program, you can skip the following paragraph.

The next chapter concerns supplements and over-the-counter medicines. I mention this because that little walk that you are reluctant to take is better for your health than any supplement in the health food store (and many of the prescription drugs on your shelf).

Additional Reading:

Natural Bypasses Can Save Lives

The Obesity/Exercise Paradox

Focus on Fitness, Not Fatness

The Big Fat Truth

ଙ୍ଚ-ଙ୍ଚ-ଙ୍ଚ-ଙ୍ଚ-ଙ୍ଚ

10 WTF Exercise Rules You Can Ignore

Walk 10,000 steps every day! Drink 8 glasses of water every day! Work out for 30 minutes every day! 100 crunches every day will shrink belly fat! And never forget – no pain, no gain! WTF?

Okay, I'll stop. The Internet is overrun with WTF (Way Too Foolish) exercise rules; my Google search found so many dopey ones that I began to giggle uncontrollably. I chose 10 of the worst and then quit – readers who haven't understood the basic concept by now are S*L*O*W*-*L*E*A*R*N*E*R*S. Here's the good news: the rules below are very popular, but there's no reason to feel guilty if you break them. And sooner or later, you will break them all. I know I will.

1. **Walk 10,000 steps every day.** This is the latest exercise fad among the chronically neurotic. They buy Fitbits or cell phone apps or old-fashioned step counters and start religiously recording details of their daily walking activity – as if any of the data could possibly matter in twelve months. Or in twelve days. The truth: the number '10,000' was invented as part of a Japanese marketing campaign for a pedometer. In 1965.

   Don't obsess over the number of steps you take; instead, get 2-5 hours of vigorous exercise each week, both cardio and strength training, and try to walk on days when you don't exercise strenuously. If you can't, don't feel guilty. Do those simple things and you will outlive your obsessive friends.

2. **Work out for thirty minutes every day.** This concept is very common, but it is truly bad advice. The body needs to rest. All the recent studies indicate that people who exercise vigorously just 3-4 days per week live longer than people who exercise vigorously every day. I like to alternate days – to work out hard one day and then simply walk my dog the next.

3. **Spot Reducing Works.** I just devoted an entire section to this idea, so why am I repeating myself? Because some of you have already forgotten the advice. S*l*o*w*–*L*e*a*r*n*e*r*s, do not listen to your friends or trainers who tell you that crunches will reduce your belly fat. Instead, ask them to tell you how they earned their high school diplomas.

4. **No Pain, No Gain.** Remember that high school gym teacher with a face like an angry meatloaf who used to scream that if it didn't hurt, it wasn't doing you any good? Somewhere along the line,

he was overcooked. Here's the truth: if something hurts, stop doing it. A little soreness the next day is common, as muscle tissues damaged during exercise heal and grow stronger. However, treat pain as a warning signal. If it hurts, stop doing it.

5. **The Longer the Workout, the Better the Benefit.** This seems to be obvious but it does not hold up. There is a fast fallout in value after about 60 minutes, depending on the person. Tell the over-achiever in your house to take off the track shoes and take a nap.

6. **A Fitness Tracker Will Keep You Fit for Years.** Wouldn't that be nice? Unfortunately, the truth is that your new fitness app will keep you fit for a few weeks before you abandon it. As of this writing, Fitbit is the latest fad activity tracker, but by the time you read this it will probably have lost most of its market share – if it has survived. It definitely won't last – they never do. Activity trackers are like health club memberships: people pay for them, devote themselves to a healthy lifestyle for a short time, and then grow bored. If you want to stay fit for years, the motivation has to come internally, not externally.

7. **Women Shouldn't Lift Weights Because It'll Make Them Bulk Up Like a Man.** Nonsense. If a woman is healthy enough to lift weights, then she should – at any age. It's almost impossible for women to develop large muscles – they don't have enough testosterone. Women with giant, hyper-developed muscles are taking enough steroids to frighten Barry Bonds. That's the bad news. The good news is that women who strength-train regularly but do not overdo it are hot.

8. **Low-Intensity Exercise Burns More Fat than High-Intensity Exercise Does.** This is a common myth perpetuated by a deep misunderstanding of the way we burn calories – and of high school math. The truth: high-intensity exercise burns more total calories. Initially more of those calories come from stored carbs, but ultimately neither high- nor low-intensity exercise burns enough calories in a single workout to make a difference. However, as time goes by, high-intensity workouts stimulate the body to grow more muscle tissue, and that burns a few more calories 24/7.

9. **Sports drinks are essential.** This is true, but only if you exercise for an hour or more and sweat profusely. If not, stick to water. Sports drinks and gels have potassium and sodium, which you probably do not need, and sugar, which you definitely do not need. What you do need is a healthy diet, which will give you all the electrolytes you want without drinking a chemical brew from a laboratory vat.

10. **If you don't work up a sweat, don't waste your time.** Here's a thought experiment. It's January and you live in North Dakota. The temperature hasn't been above zero since August, when the lifeguard was a snowman. Most days, you exercise in snow boots. You go out for your standard two-mile run through the snow and then come home. Please answer two questions: (1) While you were running, did you work up a sweat? (2) Why the hell do you live in North Dakota?

There they are – 10 Way-Too-Foolish Exercise Rules that you never need to worry about again. And here's the best part: Do you have an annoying, too-thin, over-exercised friend who is always telling you that you have to walk 10,000 steps every day and that you should always stay hydrated and that you must do 100 crunches for a flat belly every day and do both cardio and strength training every day and that if you don't work up a sweat, none of it counts? The next time she whines that you are doing something wrong, you can look her straight in the eye, smile sagely, and say, "WTF?"

Additional Reading:

No pain, no gain?

Sports drinks are not essential

When Exercise Does More Harm Than Good

****

Chapter 8: Type 2 Diabetes and The 16-Word Diet

Type 2 Diabetes is flooding the world like a tsunami. New strains of flu named after barnyard animals get the big headlines, but diabetes is the real killer, robbing millions of their health in an agonizingly slow decline. Traditionally, the disease was seen in adults past fifty, but it has spread down to teenagers, even children.

The good news: many of us can control it without meds.

Many Suspects, No Answers

Many possible causes of the unexpected epidemic are being investigated: food additives, viruses, an unhealthy mix of bacteria in the gut, environmental agents, fructose, etc., but as yet there are no confirmed answers. There are probably several causes, working separately or together; regardless, Type 2 Diabetes can be prevented, postponed or even reversed. It is the first worldwide epidemic that can be controlled by most sufferers without drugs or surgery: most cases can be managed for decades with simple changes in lifestyle.

Irrespective of the cause, one dismal fact is guaranteed: if you are an adult past forty, you have a one-in-three chance of becoming diabetic. If you are Black, Latino, or Jewish, your chances are even worse (blame your genes). However, that depressing statistic is countered by encouraging but often overlooked news: the same lifestyle changes that lower your chances of T2D will also lower your chances of heart attack or stroke. And no, you do not need to spend the rest of your life pumping iron and struggling with a low-fat diet that keeps you hungry all day. You can help yourself stay healthy, while feeling (and eating!) better than ever.

How T2D Begins

T2D incubates long before glucose levels begin rising in the blood, when the body slowly becomes resistant to insulin. Insulin's main job is to move glucose from the blood into cells, where it is used for energy or stored for future needs. But often, the body begins to use the hormone inefficiently. That condition, called insulin resistance, is the precursor to Type 2 Diabetes. The beta cells of the pancreas have to produce more and more of the hormone to keep blood glucose levels normal.

Gradually, the insulin-producing beta cells wear out and die, setting the stage for rising blood glucose, prediabetes and diabetes. The causes remain controversial, but one thing is clear: sedentary people with diets high in sugar are very likely to get Type 2 Diabetes. (For a detailed understanding of Type 2 Diabetes and how too much fructose can cause you to become diabetic, I recommend Fat Chance, by Dr. Robert Lustig. I've mentioned his two books several times, in small part because his co-author, Cindy Gershen, is a friend and in large part because his book nicely complements this one. Gershen hones in on the science of one significant cause of obesity and I focus on improving the habits and actions of the obese. You should understand both.)

In a recent New York Times column, Jane Brody wrote, "In 2012, Type 2 Diabetes accounted for $245 billion in health care expenses, about one in five health care dollars. Among its serious complications are heart disease, stroke, kidney damage, nerve damage, eye disease (which can lead to blindness), foot damage (which can lead to amputations) and hearing loss." All that suffering, even though most cases of Type 2 Diabetes can be prevented or postponed easily.

Type 2 Diabetes kills incrementally, with changes so subtle that people often do not notice until it is too late. During the 1980s, I watched as it killed my father in exquisitely small slices, robbing him of his manhood, and then his dignity, and then the use of his limbs and, ultimately, the use of his brain. The disease killed him, and caring for him almost killed my mother.

We have learned a great deal since then; in the future, what happened to my parents should not happen to any of us. Today, most patients with T2D can easily put off its ill effects for years or decades. However, they need to understand how to minimize the medicines they take and what will happen if they do not.

The Solution

The solution is well known: diet and exercise. Specifically, it's The 16-Word Diet™. I'm serious. The diet recommends reasonable portions, fresh, healthy foods, and frequent exercise, and it can be a lifesaver. It is the simplest solution to a major health problem imaginable.

Unfortunately, few people are willing to make even that minimal effort.

Given the choice between eating something that tastes good today and having their feet amputated tomorrow, or between passing on the sweets today and having a good sex life tomorrow, they say, "To Hell with my feet and my sex life!"

I will never understand this attitude. If this sounds insulting, I don't apologize. I was talking directly to every healthy person who is sedentary and has a poor diet. The good news is that diabetes can be prevented; however, you must take the first step. That first step isn't with a pill or shot; it is with yourself. You must take charge of your own health, because no doctor can do what you will not do for yourself. Taking charge is extremely simple; just make microscopic changes to your life every day, so that a year from now you will be living a healthier lifestyle.

My father and brother both became diabetic while in their forties; in addition to killing my father, the disease turned my brother into an invalid. I was diagnosed as having Type 2 Diabetes in the 1990s, also while in my forties, but I have yet to take my first pill or shot. My diabetes has not progressed; I control it with the 16-Word Diet and by carefully monitoring the meds that every doc tries to give me. Doctors are human, too, and often they take the easy way out. Please note that I'm not giving medical advice here or anywhere else – ask your doctor for his opinion.

Avoid T2D Meds or Try to Get Off Them

Most T2D patients take an escalating medley of drugs. Unfortunately, drugs just postpone the inevitable: a slow, painful death at a relatively young age, a death robbed of all dignity. People who rely on pills and refuse to live a healthier lifestyle will gradually need higher doses, and then stronger medicines, and ultimately, shots of insulin – if they live long enough. People who manage their disease with diet and exercise need fewer meds or no meds at all. As a result, they live longer, healthier, happier lives. The choice is not complicated.

A footnote to the above paragraph: many people are diagnosed with T2D when the real problem is a reaction to prescription or over-the-counter drugs. For example, diuretics are given freely to cardiac patients. Unfortunately, they are notorious for raising blood sugar levels; many patients taken off the drugs will slowly return to normal blood sugar levels.

How T2D Can Be Prevented, Postponed, or Controlled

Diabetes can be prevented, postponed, or controlled if you take charge of your treatment. Be active, not passive. For example:

- Many medicines and supplements can be a problem. Check these incomplete lists of **prescription drugs, supplements**, and **vitamins** known to raise blood sugar. Also, ask your pharmacist.

- If you have diabetes, look up every drug that you put into your body. Ask Google: "Can (drug name) increase blood sugar?" If the answer is yes, ask your doctor if you can reduce or eliminate the med with a better lifestyle. A different prescription should be a distant second choice.

- Be honest. Many patients do not tell their doctors about the supplements they take; they are afraid they will be told to stop. Apparently, these patients trust the opinion of a high school dropout working as a minimum-wage clerk in the local General Nutrition Store over the opinion of a highly trained doctor.

- If you are taking any over-the-counter product, including herbs or energy drinks, stop for a month. I promise you will not be hospitalized. See if your blood sugar improves. If it does, toss your supplements into the nearest dumpster.

- If you drink fruit juice, even fresh from your juicer, stop. Fresh juice tastes great but it is a disaster for diabetics. The general rule: apples are healthy; apple juice is unhealthy; apple pie is poison.

- Most important, follow *The 16-Word Diet*.

For many of us, *The 16-Word Diet* can help control T2D for years – even decades. Taking pills sounds easier but it isn't: over time your dosage will increase, you will be prescribed ever-stronger drugs, and the quality of your life will slowly slide downhill. The three rules offer a wonderful alternative: they will help you feel better, look better, and maintain a better sex life.

Please chose the best joke to end this chapter. I want to watch a ball game:

- Better sex. It's a great plan for the future, and it didn't come from a high school dropout working at General Nutrition.
- If those three things don't motivate you, move to a state in which recreational marijuana is legal.

The American Diabetes Association offers a simple, seven-question test to help people assess their risk; it can be found at www.diabetes.org. Important factors include a family history of the disease, prior gestational diabetes, being overweight or obese, physical inactivity and older age.

****

Just one section in this chapter. No lists of ten worst anythings, and no jokes until the end. The topic of Type 2 Diabetes is so important, and the first line of defense for most sufferers is so simple, that I wanted to isolate them into their own chapter. Obviously, there is a great deal more that T2D sufferers should learn, but I wanted to keep this chapter short and focused. Again, remember that I am not advising you to discontinue any of your prescription drugs and join a gym; I am simply suggesting that a better lifestyle is the most important change people with T2D can make if the goal is a long, healthy life.

Chapter 9: Supplements

Do You Need Supplements?

America's latest health food obsession is: replacing fresh foods with processed supplements. I'm serious.

The craze began with juicers, which are to fine dining what organ grinders are to fine music, and then entered commercial laboratories, where unregulated foods and chemicals are turned into vitamins, minerals, and protein powders by workers not qualified to put cat food into cans. Regardless, many people wash down their unregulated vitamin pills with unregulated protein drinks, which they make by casually tossing scoops of something that smells like powdered guppy into a juicer. What are they thinking?

Apparently, not much.

The 18-Word Diet?

The 16 Words are, of course:

1. Eat reasonable portions of fresh, healthy foods.

2. Avoid processed foods and sugars.

3. Get regular, vigorous exercise.

Sometimes I think I should add a fourth line: Calm Down.

People worry so much about getting proper nutrition that they overdose on expensive, unnecessary supplements. However, if you stick with The 16 Words, you can save your money. Even better, you can stop drinking things that taste like stale seaweed. Just eat a variety of fresh, healthy foods and avoid processed foods and sugar. Who would argue with that?

Apparently, many people would. Health-conscious people are eagerly eating... substances whose ingredients may once have been food before they were processed and, months later, ended up in a smoothie. Remember reading horror stories about how Frito-Lay would pulverize a perfectly good potato, stir in a variety of chemicals, form it into artificial 'chips', fry it, and then sell it as **Pringles**? Those were the good old days.

Today, intelligent people who are horrified at the idea of eating genetically modified foods will merrily dump a variety of unregulated protein boosters, vitamins, and herbal extracts into a juicer, toss in some fruits and vegetables, and then blend everything together into a fine Pringle-esque mash. However, most of the supplements they add are not regulated by any government agency; manufacturers can legally sell almost anything and call it a 'food supplement'. They can sell a bottle of ground turtle droppings and call it Ochre Aquadust, an exotic name I made up 30 seconds ago, and not much can be done to stop them. More realistically, they can use ingredients made in China, which have not been tested for, say, lead.

The worst part: those health-conscious, GMO-shunning, Ochre Aquadust-swilling consumers are not dumb teenagers who can't stop following the crowd; they are smart, well-educated adults who can't stop following the crowd. And if the crowd is gleefully gobbling turtle-crap smoothies, many smart, well-educated consumers will say, "Yum!!"

Love Your Juicer?

Before I go further, a word for those of you who love your juicers. Remember that organ grinder I mentioned earlier? A man who dresses like a gypsy and spends his days publicly cranking his organ while his monkey begs for pocket change is producing delightful carnival music that I do not want to hear very often. Similarly, juicers crank out delicious drinks that I do not want to consume very often, even if the juicer comes with a free monkey who stuffs bananas into the hopper. Like organ grinders, juicers are fun, but best enjoyed infrequently. If you insist on having them frequently, be sure to include all the pulp – it is essential for health.

Two Basic Types of Supplements

There are protein supplements and there are vitamin, mineral, and/or herbal (nutrient) supplements. Most protein promoters swear they use a magic protein that is better than anyone else's magic protein, and most nutrient promoters use a magic extract of a South American herb you never knew existed but which the promoter swears is necessary to save your life.

I remember the 1970s, when spirulina (dried blue green algae) was promoted as a way to lose weight, build muscle, improve cardiac function, blah, blah, blah. Years have gone by, and I have yet to read about a single emergency room doctor emerging from a single operating room to proclaim, "If he hadn't been taking spirulina, we would have lost him." Until that happens, I'm not swallowing spirulina or anything else that looks like powdered leprechaun. Remember that, the next time a brilliant marketing campaign tries to seduce you into buying an herb that you never heard of but that you are suddenly convinced you desperately need.

Protein boosters are useful if you are recovering from a serious illness or training hard; otherwise, you may not need them. The best way to get protein is to eat a variety of healthy sources (fish, meat, chicken, eggs, tofu, cottage cheese, etc.) and to avoid processed protein (hot dogs, beef jerky, etc.). Follow Rule 1.

That said, if your life is in an extremely busy phase and sometimes you do not have the time to cook properly for yourself, a quality protein supplement is greatly superior to fast food. Having a protein supplement a few times a week as a meal replacement is fine, as long as there isn't too much added sugar (or honey, etc.).

Vitamin and Mineral Supplements

Vitamin and mineral supplements are not normally needed by healthy people who have several portions of varied fruits and vegetables per day. Many supplements are made with unregulated, potentially dangerous herbs. Often, they are overloaded with unnecessary antioxidants, so that they can brag about them on the labels.

Complete meal replacements are essentially protein boosters with added fat and carbohydrates. The market for those products is stagnant, so manufacturers have tried to expand their markets by appealing to people who are too busy to eat. I'm serious. One product has a video with a solemn-sounding voice-over saying, "You can take the time you'd normally spend preparing, eating and cleaning up after meals, and put that time into other areas of your life."

It's a great sales pitch for people with lives as empty as that monkey on an organ grinder's tether. If you want to have an occasional meal replacement as a quick, balanced meal, wonderful. If you plan to live on them and only them for the next three months, get a better plan.

Here's a simple suggestion: instead of spending a fortune on dubious supplements, buy a new pair of walking shoes. Use them to take your dog on longer walks. That will improve your health better than any herbal supplement can.

❦❦❦❦❦

Most Herbal Supplements Do Not Contain Herbs. Do Yours?

Here's some unsurprising news: roughly four out of five herbal supplements do not contain the herbs listed on their labels. And yes, that probably includes your favorite brand. After independent testing, the New York State Attorney General and three other AGs sent <u>cease-and-desist letters</u> to four major retailers, asking how they verify the ingredients in their herbal supplements. (Hint: they don't.) Some examples from the 2015 complaint:

- **GNC:** Ginkgo biloba from GNC contains rice, asparagus, citrus, and spruce, but no ginkgo biloba. GNC Echinacea did not have any echinacea but it did have rice.

- **Walgreen's:** Garlic supplements from Walgreens contain no garlic. However, you can buy their ginseng supplement, which has lots of garlic – but no ginseng.

- **Walmart:** Ginkgo biloba from Walmart contains... powdered vegetation. Radish, houseplants, and wheat, but no ginkgo biloba.

- **Target:** St. John's wort and valerian root from Target contain no medicinal herbs of any sort, only rice, beans, peas, and carrots.

Hmm... rice, beans, peas, carrots, garlic, asparagus, citrus, wheat, and radish. And powdered houseplants? Sounds like a side dish from a bad Chinese restaurant. You may be spending $100 per month on someone's leftovers.

Can You Ever Trust Supplements and Vitamins?

After extensive independent testing found massive fraud in the herbal supplements sold by four major retailers, the New York State Attorney General sent cease-and-desist letters to GNC, Target, Walgreens, and

Walmart. However, if your favorite store or website is not on the list, you are not safe. It only means that your favorite products weren't tested.

It gets worse. If you proudly purchase from a high-end vitamin and supplement manufacturer, perhaps one that guarantees it manufactures its own products in a pristine laboratory using nothing but organic herbs and spring water, then you are proudly buying from a pristine lab that may not exist. Your pills are probably coming from the same unregulated factories in China, India, or Utah that the big box stores buy from; your high-end manufacturer is lying to you at a high level. Personally, I think that all herbal supplements should be packaged in white cardboard Chinese take-out containers. At least that would be honest.

Okay – you want me to back up. China, India, and… *Utah*? Yes, the great majority of vitamins produced in this country are made in Utah, and they are not regulated. In 1994, Utah Senator Orrin Hatch protected his largest political donors by pushing a law through Congress that exempted vitamins and supplements from the F.D.A.'s strict approval process for prescription drugs. He also blocked countless bills that would have protected us from his donors, mainly snake oil manufacturers employing sleazy whores. Wait! I'm sorry – I meant to type 'well-paid lobbyists'.

The results were predictable: manufacturers now use the least expensive ingredients available, regardless of what the label says. For example, Walmart supplements that claim to be wheat-free and gluten-free were found to be loaded with wheat or pine – dangerous for people with allergies. Worse, products from other retailers had traces of legumes, which might hospitalize people with hypersensitivity to peanuts. Orrin Hatch's refusal to regulate the vitamin and supplement industry has allowed it to sell poison and call it pixie dust.

If Your Herbal Supplements Are Fake, What Should You Do?

First, don't panic. If you were taking, say, valerian root as a helpful sleep aid but the pills were actually filled with powdered rice, then you do not need a sleep aid. That's good news. Second, if you have been taking supplements to compensate for an unhealthy diet, then stop eating an unhealthy diet. No vitamin complex or herbal supplement can improve your health or control your weight the way that common sense can: eat reasonable portions of fresh, healthy foods, avoid processed foods and sugars, and get regular, vigorous exercise. I hope that sounds familiar. (If it doesn't, then you have just discovered that you are a S*l*o*w*- *L*e*a*r*n*e*r. **Please return to page 1 and start reading again. When you get back here, give yourself a happy face.**☺

More important, don't automatically reject medical doctors and prescription drugs while bravely saying, "I don't trust Western Medicine." That's wellness by popular mythology, not by logic or wisdom. I have no love for Big Pharma, but I trust the FDA more than I trust unregulated discount vitamin websites that use pretty labels to mask sham products. Also, I trust regulated prescription drug manufacturers more than I trust unregulated supplement manufacturers, who, with no oversight, can put dehydrated school cafeteria lunch leftovers into a capsule and sell it as organic herbal magic.

Before you say, "That's obvious," think of all the money well-meaning people have spent on bottles of magic herbal supplements that are stuffed with rice, asparagus, citrus, wheat, radish, beans, peas, carrots, and houseplants but no herbs. Maybe Walmart's should start selling its supplements in white cardboard take-out containers.

****

Despite my merry rant, some supplements have merit. Probiotics are a wonderful if confusing example.

ๆ๛๛๛๛

Should You Be Taking Probiotics?

Probiotics fascinate me. Everybody wants to take them but no one knows why.

Probiotics are one of the few dietary products that offer legitimate benefits to most people. Sold without a prescription, they have grown steadily in popularity for more than two decades and are now surging. Unlike the vast majority of over-the-counter supplements, probiotics work: they can relieve many health problems. However, before you run to the health food store or begin mainlining yogurt, there are several things you should know: what probiotics can do, which brands you can trust, which specific probiotics will treat different conditions, and (most important) what the hell are probiotics?

I get strange questions.

Q: "If I take probiotics, can I eat more carbs?"
A: *Yes, but you will get fatter.*

Q: "Will probiotics help my diet?"
A: *No. Dieting will help your diet.*

Q: "Will Probiotics help my chronic explosive diarrhea?"
A: *Maybe. Now, never write to me again.*

What are Probiotics?

According to *New York Times* Wellness Expert Jane Brody, "**Probiotics** are defined by the World Health Organization as 'live micro-organisms which, when administered in adequate amounts, confer a health benefit on the host.' Their benefits range from relieving infection-caused diarrhea, inflammatory bowel diseases, and irritable bowel syndrome to helping patients with asthma, allergy, and Type 1 diabetes."

Translation: Probiotics are bugs that make your gut healthier.

Probiotics, Prebiotics and Synbiotics

Two other terms complete the picture: prebiotics and synbiotics. **Prebiotics** are non-digestible carbohydrates that stimulate the growth of probiotic organisms in the gut. They are found in oats, wheat, bananas, onions, garlic, leeks, asparagus, soybeans, honey, and artichokes. **Synbiotics,** a combination of prebiotics and probiotics, are found in yogurt and kefir, fermented foods like pickles and some cheeses, and in some supplements. Yes, some supplements are actually good for us.

A quick overview: probiotics are beneficial bacteria that live in your body and offer a health benefit. Prebiotics feed the little beasts. Synbiotics are foods that contain both prebiotics and probiotics and still taste good, which apparently is not impossible.

Northern Europeans frequently consume probiotics because of their tradition of eating foods fermented with bacteria, such as yogurt and cheese. Probiotic-laced beverages are also big business in Japan. However, probiotic foods have lagged in the United States while probiotic supplements have grown rapidly. Tell Americans there is a health issue and we will try to fix it with a pill.

Before you take a probiotic, decide what you want it to do for your health. Then, Google your symptom and the word 'probiotic'. For example, Google "will probiotics help Grandpa with his gas?" After you find the appropriate bacteria strain (or yeast strain), find a supplement that contains that specific organism. Just be careful; if you go to your local health food store and purchase a beautifully labeled package of pills, you will have no way of knowing if the pills contain probiotics or cow pie. And even if they do have billions of probiotic beasties ready to populate your intestines, you don't know if you are getting the strain you are looking for to treat your particular problem. Cross your fingers.

Why are things so confusing? First, no government agency regularly tests supplements to see what they contain. Second, there is **no legal definition** of 'Probiotics'. Someone could legally sell crunchy wafers of Mr. Magic's All-Natural Probiotic Moon Dust and safely make millions of dollars.

Will Probiotics Help You Lose Weight?

Legitimate researchers have proven that many different strains of bacteria, fungi, and yeasts can have a positive impact on your gastrointestinal tract. Unfortunately, they cannot help you lose weight – sorry. The only studies that showed positive weight loss results were small, short-term projects sponsored by companies that sell probiotics – hardly an objective crowd. Independent studies have shown that the bacterial strains under review did not help dieters.

Several supplements and yogurt drinks have been evaluated properly and found to be excellent aids to digestion. Culturelle contains Lactobacillus GG; Align contains Bifidobacterium infantis 35624 (also marketed as Bifantis). Both are recommended for people taking lengthy courses of antibiotics. VSL#3 was specifically designed for the dietary management of ulcerative colitis, an ileal pouch, and irritable bowel syndrome.

The probiotics marketplace can be confusing. Decide what your needs are, look online, find the specific strain of bacteria or yeast that helps your problem, then find a food that contains it. As of this writing (2016), select between Align, Culturelle, or VSL#3. For about $0.75 a day, you will know exactly what you are getting.

Additional Reading:

These websites have valuable information about probiotics:

- **Health benefits of taking probiotics (Harvard)**

- **Consumer Reports – Probiotics can help prevent dangerous infections**

- **Prebiotics, probiotics and digestive health.**

ৼৼৼৼৼ

Do Fish-Oil Supplements Work?

Fish-oil supplements may be the most popular OTC product introduced in the last 25 years. Loaded with omega-3 fatty acids, they are said to help reduce heart disease and stroke, lower blood pressure, ease arthritis pain, reduce triglycerides, slow the development of arterial plaque, etc. People all over the world take them every day. Thousands of doctors prescribe them to patients. But do fish-oil supplements really work?

No one knows for sure. The latest studies are... spotty.

The Fish-Oil Story Began with a Bad Guess

About fifty years ago, scientists began to study the Inuit people, groups of indigenous peoples inhabiting the Arctic regions of Greenland, Canada, and Alaska. The Inuit lived almost exclusively on a high saturated fat diet, but their incidence of heart disease and stroke was quite low.

According to the _New York Times_, as the Inuit people spread across the Arctic thousands of years ago, they developed one of the most extreme diets on Earth. They didn't farm fruits, vegetables or grains and there weren't many wild plants to forage, aside from an occasional patch of berries on the tundra. For the most part, the Inuit ate what they could hunt: mainly whales, seals and fish.

In the 1970s, Danish researchers who were studying Inuit metabolism proposed that the omega-3 fatty acids found in fish were protective. This eventually led to the recommendation that Westerners eat more fish to help prevent heart disease. Gradually, millions of people added fish or fish-oil supplements to their daily diet; Americans now spend over $1 billion on fish oil in pill form. But according to the latest research and studies, the pill form doesn't seem to work.

Forty Years Later, Better Studies Emerged

One early clue came from the **National Institutes of Health** website, which states,

- There has been substantial research on supplements of omega-3s, particularly in seafood and fish oil, and heart disease. The findings of individual studies have been inconsistent. In 2012, two combined analyses of the results did not find convincing evidence these omega-3s protect against heart disease.

- Evidence suggests that seafood rich in omega-3 fatty acids should be included in a heart-healthy diet. However, omega-3s in supplement form have not been shown to protect against heart disease.

- Epidemiological studies done more than 30 years ago noted relatively low death rates due to cardiovascular disease in Eskimo populations with high seafood consumption. Since then, much research has been done on seafood and heart disease. The results provide moderate evidence that people who eat seafood at least once a week are less likely to die of heart disease than those who rarely or never eat seafood.

Translation: Eating fish is probably good for us. Taking fish oil pills is probably not.

But didn't Danish researchers prove that fish oil works? That it keeps heart disease and stroke low among the Inuit in the Arctic? No. The standards for studies were laxer during the 1970s. (A lot of things were laxer during the Seventies. I miss those days.) The Danish researchers merely found that heart disease is low among the Inuit, and then hypothesized that fish oil was the protective agent.

They published their theory as an educated guess, and slowly but surely it became gospel. A number of studies confirmed the theory, but in retrospect the studies were poorly conducted or poorly analyzed. Also, fish oil manufacturing was substandard.

The Answer Might Be in Inuit Genes

A study recently published in the journal *Science* reported that the ancestors of the Inuit evolved unique genetic adaptations for metabolizing omega-3s and other fatty acids. Those gene variants had drastic effects on Inuit bodies, reducing their heights and weights and allowing them to thrive on a very high-fat diet with few vegetables or fruit.

Rasmus Nielsen, a geneticist at the University of California, Berkeley, and an author of the new study, said that this discovery raised questions about whether omega-3 fats really were protective against heart disease and stroke, despite the decades of advocacy. "The same diet may have different effects on different people," he said.

The researchers found several genetic variants at different locations in the Inuit genome that occurred quite frequently compared with genomes from people in Europe or China. Some of the variations produce enzymes that help regulate the different fats in our bloodstreams, including omega-3 fatty acids. One specific gene variant was present in almost every Inuit in the study; it is far less common in other populations. About 25% of Chinese people have it and just 2% of Europeans do.

People with two copies of the Inuit gene had different blood levels of fatty acids than people without them. Also, it is probable that their gut bacteria evolved to be very different from the standard Western assortment, although the effects haven't been studied (to my knowledge).

The Inuit seem to have evolved a mechanism to bring blood levels of fatty acids back into a healthy balance. Dr. Nielsen and his colleagues are planning to investigate the long-term health effects of the gene variants they've found, to learn why some of us metabolize fats more effectively than others, and why omega-3s haven't been the heart panacea we all hoped for.

Should You Continue to Take Fish-Oil Supplements?

So – if you take fish oil, what should you do? According to NIH, you should eat fish every week and not rely on the pills lessening your chances of heart disease or stroke; they probably will not. However, if fish-oil supplements help you with arthritis pain, or if your blood pressure has gone down since you started taking them, or if fish oil has another beneficial effect on your body, why stop? Buy them from the most reputable source you can find, and stay healthy – if the particular brand you purchase actually has sufficient omega-3s from fish oil, and is not rancid: From *The New York Times*: "Despite their popularity, some studies have found that roughly three-quarters of fish oil supplements on the market do not contain the amount of omega-3 fatty acids advertised on their labels. Some have also found that fish oil supplements are prone to becoming rancid."

Are other supplements equally questionable? That's what this chapter is about. That said, let's look at one that sounds promising.

৯৯৯৯৯

Is Inulin-Propionate Ester the Miracle Diet Drug We've Been Waiting for?

An interesting question. First, get used to that unwieldy chemical name; in a few years, you're going to see it everywhere. Worldwide headlines are screaming that inulin propionate ester actually works, reducing not just our appetites but our food cravings. I've craved pizza non-stop since 1968, so I researched this topic carefully – almost joyfully. Surprisingly, my conclusion is:

Maybe.

There are actually three stories here: the promising things that scientists are learning about inulin propionate ester, the distortions from the media, and how disgracefully easy it is to buy it as an over-the-counter supplement. First, the science.

A Legitimate Diet Drug or Just Another Scam?

Inulin PE may be the real thing. <u>In a study published in July, 2016,</u> scientists from Imperial College London and the University of Glasgow asked 20 healthy, non-obese men to consume a milkshake that either contained inulin-propionate ester or one of its precursors, a natural fiber called inulin. Trace amounts of inulin are found in sugar beets, asparagus, onions, wheat, etc., but you can't eat enough to make a difference.

Previous studies have shown that bacteria in the gut release a chemical called propionate when they digest inulin. Propionate can signal the brain to reduce your appetite, and the inulin-propionate ester supplement apparently releases much more propionate in the intestines than inulin alone. (Note to people who would refuse to add propionate to their foods because it is a chemical: Learn something.)

After drinking the milkshakes, the participants in the current study underwent an MRI scan, where they were shown pictures of various low- or high-calorie foods such as salad, fish and vegetables or chocolate, cake and pizza.

The team found that when volunteers drank the milkshake containing inulin-propionate ester, they had less activity in the 'reward-centers' in their brains. Remarkably, this only occurred when looking at the high-calorie foods. The volunteers also had to rate how appealing they found the foods; when they drank milkshakes with the inulin-propionate ester supplement, they rated the high-calorie foods as less appealing than when they drank shakes that only contained inulin.

All the Hype Is Based on Two Small Studies

A 2013 research study by the same team found that overweight volunteers who added an inulin-propionate ester supplement to their food every day gained less weight over six months than did volunteers who added only inulin to their meals.

In a second part of the study, published in the July edition of the *American Journal of Clinical Nutrition*, volunteers were given a bowl of pasta with tomato sauce, and asked to eat as much as they liked. When participants drank the inulin-propionate ester milkshake, they ate 10 per cent less pasta than when they drank the milkshake that contained inulin alone.

Professor Gary Frost, senior author of the study, said: "We know that adults gain between 0.3 and 0.8 kilos (0.66-1.75 pounds) a year on average, and there's a real need for new strategies that can prevent this. Molecules like propionate stimulate the release of gut hormones that control appetite, but you need to eat huge amounts of fiber to achieve a strong effect. We wanted to find a more efficient way to deliver propionate to the gut. This small, proof-of-principle study shows encouraging signs that supplementing one's diet with the ingredient we've developed prevents weight gain in overweight people."

"Our previous findings showed that people who ate this ingredient gained less weight – but we did not know why. This study is filling in a missing bit of the jigsaw – this supplement can decrease activity in brain areas associated with food reward at the same time as reducing the amount of food they eat."

Should You Ask Your Doctor About Inulin-Propionate Ester?

Not yet. No one knows for sure if it is safe and effective, or if it has a side effect that hasn't been seen yet. Most of the articles breathlessly describing inulin-propionate ester as a miracle ignored a basic fact: everything we know about it is based on a few small, uncontrolled studies meant only to see if larger studies are warranted. The researchers tested 20 healthy, non-obese men – no women, no obese people, no one with heart disease or diabetes, just 20 healthy guys, a group easily distracted by any bright and shiny object in the room. Such as a nurse carrying a milkshake.

Also, the 2013 study was specifically designed to show that ordinary adults, who tend to gain a small amount of weight every year, would not gain if they regularly took inulin PE. No one tested obese people to see if the chemical could actually help them lose weight. That's a very different question. Before scientists can claim that inulin PE is a legitimate, low-risk diet aid, they will need to conduct lengthy, well-funded studies. Basic science.

Of course, basic science didn't stop the Shameless Headline Whores from making false claims. Headlines claiming that Inulin-Propionate Ester Is a Miracle Diet Drug are sprouting faster than marijuana plants in Colorado.

The following headlines are real — you can Google them:

- Scientists Have Found a Supplement That Can Switch Off Junk Food Cravings

- Revolutionary Fiber Milkshake Could Help Dieters Shed the Pounds by Switching Off Cravings for Junk Food

- Inulin-Propionate Ester Ingredient Will Make You Feel Fuller

- Scientists Can Now Switch Off Your High-Calorie Cravings

- Inulin-Propionate Ester May Be the Key to Solving the World's Obesity Crisis

- Inulin-Propionate Ester Replaces Minoxidil as World's Top Selling Baldness Cure!

Okay, the last headline was fake. But before you get cranky, think about this: Is my fake headline less ridiculous than the five real headlines above it?

Should You Take Inulin PE Supplements?

Not yet. The product is easy to find online and in health food stores, but I recommend against it until more studies are published — solidly conducted studies involving thousands of subjects. First, the present studies are tiny and flawed. Second, there's an important reason to not take the drug: you have no way to know what is in the bottle. It might be the real thing; it might be cornstarch. And please don't think that your favorite vitamin and supplement manufacturer is trustworthy; it is not. The packaging may have a beautiful, reassuring, enticing appearance, but so do shameless whores.

You are welcome to try your luck, but be careful. (That's the advice that the captain of a ship will give to sailors going on leave, and it's not a coincidence.)

****

It's difficult to leave the topic of sailors and shameless whores (so many jokes, so little time). Regardless, let's look at a few utterly worthless supplements that people are wasting their money on when they could be buying copies of *The 16-Word Diet* for their friends.

ৡৡৡৡৡ

10 Worst Supplements of the Decade – So Far

Testosterone boosters, detox cleanses, herbal cures for incurable diseases, energy drinks, herbal diet pills, Alzheimer's cures, and worse. Unregulated 'miracle' supplements keep crawling out of dark spaces like cockroaches, coated with outlandish claims, supported by junk science, and protected by ineffective laws passed by corrupt politicians. People throw billions of dollars at them every year, not to exterminate them but to buy them (both the useless cures and the useless politicians).

Here are a few 'miracle supplements' that I find particularly offensive:

1. The Ten-Day Green Smoothie Cleanse: Buying a cleanse for your intestines makes as much sense as buying shampoo if you are bald. And believe me, I know bald.

2. Plexus Slim: No, Plexus Slim was not the name of the muscular street fighter in "Sons of Anarchy". Plexus Slim is a typical weight-loss scam; a high-protein diet washed down with magic Plexus Slim juice and enchanted Plexus Slim capsules. The claims on its website are so preposterous, Dr. Oz wouldn't believe them. And he still thinks that Peter Pan is real. Or maybe he thinks he is Peter Pan.

3. 'Natural' Testosterone Boosters: Men past forty, pay attention: If you are losing your sex drive, you will not find it in a magic bottle of pills. I can legally go to the zoo, scrape up whatever the monkeys are throwing out of their cages, bottle it, and claim that it "Reinforces Male Performance". Why? Because the claim "Reinforces Male Performance" has no legal meaning. I just made it up. People selling 'testosterone boosters' do the same thing.

   Over-the-counter testosterone supplements are fakes, and many are dangerous. What works? Seeing a qualified doctor. Also, you should lose weight, exercise, get plenty of sleep, and follow The 16 Words. Adult behavior is the best way to 'Reinforce Male Performance'.

4. Omnitrition: This sounds like a new X-Box game, but it's just Bottled Bullflop. ('Magic in a bottle' isn't sufficiently insulting.)

The company claims to be selling a weight loss hormone called hCG, which is produced by pregnant women; however, hCG is illegal in the United States (and ineffective for weight loss). Omnitrition is either selling a bottle of colored water that's labeled as hCG, or it's selling homeopathic hCG, which would be a bottle of clear water that's labeled with claims too stupid to rise to the level of ordinary bull droppings.

5. The 17-Day Diet: This book pretends to be a protein-centered eating plan, but it's just a clever way to peddle their own brand of probiotics. Probiotics can be wonderful; however, despite intense research, we still know almost nothing about which specific gut bacteria can aid weight loss.

6. Red Bull, Monster, Rock Star, Five-Hour Energy: Do you drink any of these 'energy drinks' frequently? What the hell are you thinking?

7. Chinese Herbal Supplements: To repeat, any supplement made in China is potentially dangerous. There is no way to know if it contains beneficial herbs or goat cud. Recently, the FDA recalled a range of Chinese herbal supplements produced by Herbal Science International, Inc. after they were found to contain ephedrine (a powerful stimulant), other dangerous chemicals, and – seriously – human placenta. Whether or not consuming human placenta constitutes cannibalism is subject to debate, but either way, scientists say that eating it can transmit blood-borne diseases like hepatitis and HIV. People who buy an over-the-counter supplement made in China aren't slow learners, they have a death wish.

8. The Ten-Day Detox Diet: Detox diets are great for people who eat a lot of lead paint and asbestos shingles. If you don't, then you have nothing to detox. How do I know? Hundreds of thousands of autopsies have proven it.

9. Products that 'Prevent Alzheimer's': Sometimes, Evil is almost unnoticeable. For example, a product called "Brain Armor", sold by Amazon, Walmart, etc., claims to provide protection against Alzheimer's, dementia, stroke, and more. What's the problem?

People buy this crap instead of getting medical treatment to slow down their disease. Any product that claims it 'Supports Healthy Brain Function' or has any other effect on your brain is a scam. Sen. Claire McCaskill (D-MO), who likes to quote from Jay's Blog, has begun to challenge the biggest retailers, but her best efforts will slow down the snake oil peddlers for about six weeks.

10. Skinny Fiber: A magic formula that turns fibers extracted from three worthless weeds into Magic Weight Loss Fairy Dust. *Sprinkle it on your food and watch the pounds melt away!* Here's my idea: instead of swallowing it, why not put it in your back pocket? If Skinny Fiber really melts the pounds away, you'll never need to ask anyone if your ass looks fat.

One last point. Many of you are thinking to yourselves, "It's a shame that so many people take worthless herbal supplements. However, the herbal supplements that I take are excellent. They are made by a very trustworthy manufacturer and sold by an honorable retailer, and they keep me healthy." If you are one of those people, what part of being a S*l*o*w*-*L*e*a*r*n*e*r didn't you understand?

****

As I was writing this chapter, my wife forwarded to me the latest horror story about supplements made with dangerous ingredients. The supplements are Ayurvedic products made in India, and they are contaminated with high levels of both mercury and lead. This is a common problem with imports from India and China. If you are one of those people who proudly brags that you are 'tired of Western Medicine' and prefer 'Ancient Eastern Traditions', please do yourself a favor. Go back to the last section and reread the part about "shameless whores".

Additional Reading

Appetite for Diet Supplements Benefits Few, Experts Say

Fish oil pills: A $1.2 billion industry built, so far, on empty promises

Diet, not pills, may still be the best bet for brain power

Summary

Okay – now that I've had some fun, I should again stress a basic point: There is nothing wrong with taking a basic, comprehensive multi-vitamin and mineral supplement. We all live busy lives, and sometimes it is impossible to eat fresh, healthy foods and to avoid processed foods and sugars. A multi-vitamin might be a smart move. Maybe. Just remember that it can never be a substitute for long-term healthy eating. Also, multi-vitamin and mineral supplements, like other supplements, are often manufactured in Utah, where the health standards are much higher than they are in China, Vietnam, etc. I am not saying that supplements made in Utah will make you healthy; I'm just saying they won't kill you.

In general, I'm not a fan of taking high doses of specific vitamins or minerals – that approach to nutrition has no balance. It's like overinflating one tire on your car while leaving the other three underinflated. A good, general-purpose multi-vitamin and mineral supplement is fine if you can't get enough from your diet, but taking mega-doses of specific vitamins or minerals makes no sense. Worse, it's potentially dangerous.

Probiotics are excellent for your health, and if you cannot get enough in foods (i.e., if you are taking antibiotics), then probiotic supplements are an excellent choice, along with yogurt, kefir, etc. Fish oil capsules remain on the endangered list; they may survive as medically useful, but no one knows for sure. If you do not eat fish, they might be a good choice, but not great.

As of this writing, omega-3 supplements have been found to be useless in several studies. Foods containing omega-3 oil are very healthy, but the capsules do not work. Will that change as new studies come in? Who knows? It's just another reason to eat well and exercise.

Protein supplements can be wonderful in the right circumstances, and they make a fine *occasional* meal replacement, as long as the protein powder comes from a reliable source and doesn't make outrageous claims about 'miracle muscle-building potential' or similar nonsense.

The worst supplements are the ones that claim to be made from superfoods, or from specific plants or minerals that you never heard of. These are uniformly garbage. If you want the nutritious benefits of kale or carrots, eat kale and carrots. Don't swallow a pill that someone claims was made from dried kale or ground carrots – who knows what is really inside it? Eat fresh, healthy, unprocessed foods and your body will thank you. And so will your checkbook.

Still have your doubts? The PBS show Frontline had a powerful exposé of the supplement industry. It focused on fish oil capsules because they are so popular, but it applies to every over-the-counter vitamin, mineral, herbal supplement, etc., sold in the US. You can see it here.

That said, always listen to your doctor. There are many solid medical reasons for taking specific vitamins or minerals, and your doc is far more trustworthy than some website promising to send you bottles of magic that can cure every known disease.

Finally, do not take advice from your best friend from childhood who swears your life will improve if only you take some supplement that you never heard of, and BTW, he has several pallet-loads of the stuff in his garage. If, after reading this entire chapter, you haven't understood that the vast majority of vitamins, minerals, and supplements are overpriced and overrated, then you are the s*l*o*w*e*s*t – l*e*a*r*n*e*r in my class.

Chapter 10: Frauds, Fads, and Magic Pills

Introduction:

I'll open this chapter with a gentle, non-judgmental opinion: The Diet Industry is almost as corrupt as Congress, and almost as stupid. Okay, that was gentle, non-judgmental, and written with just a touch of sulfuric acid. But true. Facts do not matter, scientific research does not matter, and the health of the general public is ignored; what matters is money. No one cares about what keeps the money flowing, as long as it continues to flow in the right direction. Ridiculous but attractive ideas are successfully promoted despite the harm they can do to the public health, because the public loves to throw money at any loudmouth who can spout ridiculous ideas in a clear voice.

That, of course, was a description of how Congress works. The Diet Industry has more regulations than does The Congress, and ultimately it is less corrupt. Regardless, it is an eternal fountain of gold, forever replenished by desperate people looking for magic paths to create some unattainably desirable image they have of themselves.

It's Easy to Get Rich in the Diet Industry:
- Create a ridiculous new variation on a high-protein diet and write a book about it.
- Find an easy-to grow tropical weed that no one north of the Amazon Rainforest has ever heard of, and call it *"A diet miracle that melts fat in just days."*
- Swear that you have discovered a magic technique for exercising away belly fat.
- Guarantee that you have a secret way to help people lose vast amounts of weight even faster than the last liar who promised he had a secret way to help people lose vast amounts of weight.
- Write a book called *"The Diet Fairy is Real!"* (If you do, Oprah will return to TV to interview you.)

Yes, any clown can get rich in the Diet Industry if he is willing to say something disgracefully stupid but flashy. And many clowns have. (Am I jealous? Sometimes I want to go on Amazon.com and order a red foam rubber nose.)

This chapter was designed to help you spot the fraudulent diet products, diet books, and exercise scams that sprout up like weeds in the Amazon. I did my best to cover the most common scams, but be careful – it's a jungle out there.

৶৶৶৶৶

Do Cleanses Remove Toxins from Your Body?

Sometimes bad advice comes from friends or celebrity 'experts'; sometimes it comes from thin air. That's how cleansing seems to have appeared; one day it was an obsolete remedy mentioned in obscure texts about the history of medicine, along with blood-letting and leeches, and the next day it was a major topic of conversation at Starbuck's. That'll ruin your extra hot, sugar-free, double shot, half-decaf, non-fat vanilla soy, white chocolate mocha venti with light whip and extra syrup.

Cleansing has somehow become a surprisingly popular fad, which is surprising; the point of a cleanse is to give yourself diarrhea and eliminate imaginary 'toxins' from your liver and intestines, not to do something useful, like cleansing the Internet of all traces of cat videos.

The problem is that a remarkable number of wellness websites specialize in frightening people into buying worthless products to cure non-existent health problems, and they struck gold with cleanses. First, they warn you that your body is full of 'toxins', or insist that several pounds of decaying fecal material are stubbornly clinging to your intestinal walls. Next, they sell drinks and enemas that will 'purify' your body, 'cleanse' your intestines, and 'detoxify' your liver. The scammers aren't cleaning out your intestines – they are cleaning out your bank account.

Does Research Support Cleansing?

Regardless of the ominous claims made all over the Internet, cleansing is nonsense. Unscientific foolishness from the lunatic fringe. Your liver is not full of 'toxins', your intestines are not clogged with feces from 1999, and regardless of how safe, exotic, and effective the various herbs in a cleanse sound, they have neither science nor legitimate testing to support them. Every cleanse on the market consists of a semi-random mix of herbs tossed together by someone trying to make a buck, not by someone eager to polish the walls of your bowels.

There are two basic types of cleanse products, one that's taken orally and one that's administered as an enema. A typical oral cleanse will contain the usual suspects: exotic flowers, wild tree bark, and herbal extracts. It will also contain laxatives: senna, psyllium husk, etc. The laxatives do the actual 'cleansing'; the purpose of the esoteric ingredients is to impress the gullible consumer.

A typical colon cleansing solution will use water, salt, and... exotic flowers, wild tree bark, and herbal extracts. And often, detergent. I'm serious. Something has to clean you out and it won't be the wild tree bark. You can administer the enema yourself or go to a health spa and have a 'Colon Hydrotherapist' do it.

Health tip: if someone's business card says 'Colon Hydrotherapist', it's a safe bet that he did not get his certification from Harvard Medical School. That said, why would you let him shove a tube up your ass? Why would you even shake his hand?

On a related note, there are also 'juice cleanses', in which people consume nothing but fruit and vegetable juice for three days. No proteins, no fats, and no fiber for 72 hours. Just sugary juice. Do you know the difference between living on juice and living on Coca Cola and stale vitamins? Neither do I.

If you are still wavering, ask yourself why the person who taught you about juice cleanses is more qualified to give you medical advice than a Colon Hydrotherapist.

Nature Is a Brilliant Engineer

The human body is an astonishing machine just as nature designed it, and hard to improve. For example, your liver does an amazingly effective job of clearing toxins and other unwanted substances from your body, and your kidneys and your lower intestines prevent reabsorption. Nature designed your liver to 'cleanse' itself. If it didn't, you would have died long ago.

How do we know this? Because hundreds of thousands of human livers have been dissected and analyzed, and none of them contain accumulated toxins. The only exceptions: long-term alcoholics, morbidly obese people, and the poor people who died from advanced liver disease or cancer. That isn't you.

According to Wikipedia, "People who practice colon cleansing believe that accumulations of putrefied feces line the walls of the large intestine, and that these accumulations harbor parasites or pathogenic gut flora." That ancient theory was disproven over a hundred years ago, when doctors began to dissect corpses scientifically.

Since then, countless gastrointestinal tracts have been examined from living patients. The conclusion? No one accumulates 'putrefied feces' that need to be 'cleansed' from the intestines, unless he or she is near death from bowel disease. In plain English, YOU DO NOT HAVE OLD CRAP THAT NEEDS TO BE FLUSHED OUT OF YOUR INTESTINAL TRACT! If you did, it would have killed you long ago.

More truth: cleanses can be dangerous. Here is what doctors (medical doctors, not colon hydrotherapists) worry about:

- Some herbs may reduce the effectiveness of prescription drugs. (Dr. Stephen Barrett)

- Some enema preparations have been associated with kidney damage, heart attacks and electrolyte imbalances

- Improperly prepared or used equipment can cause infection or damage to the bowel.

- Frequent colon cleansing can lead to constipation and dependence on enemas.

- Cleanses may hurt the healthy balance of gut bacteria that we all need.

Do Cleanses Help People Lose Weight?

No. They do not help you lose fat. If you cleanse, you will temporarily dehydrate yourself, so you will be one or two pounds lighter. You will also temporarily empty your bowels, so that you will be another pound or two lighter. That 'weight loss' will last two or three days, and no one will see a difference. Why bother?

To me, cleansing is like a habit-forming drug. If you don't cleanse, don't start. If you have already started, then stop. Instead of spending your money on something so unnecessary, why not simply flush your money down the toilet and eliminate the unpleasant part where you get diarrhea? That way, you can spend your afternoons taking a walk or a nice nap instead of sitting on the toilet. A walk and a nap are better for your health. And your wallet.

A minor refinement: it is not physically possible for fecal material to accumulate on the walls of a healthy intestine – unless you are a member of Congress. If you are, go cleanse yourself.

Cleansing is not the only unscientific fad that impresses people. Most popular diet books gain their popularity the old-fashioned way: they were promoted by a charismatic author who touted his unscientific theories to a desperate public searching for solutions to the Obesity Problem.

****

Diet programs that only work for a few weeks and spot-reducing exercise programs that do not help people lose weight where they want to lose it are two parts of the misinformation problem. The third complicated problem concerns supplements. Do we really need them? Here's a hint: Because I run a successful diet and exercise blog, I can get all the vitamins and supplements I want at no charge if I simply write a few kind words about them. I don't take any.

Chapter 11: Closing Thoughts

I made a promise to you in the introduction and hope I kept it: I promised that this would be a unique book about weight loss – a book devoted to helping you build a healthier life, not devoted to selling you enchanted diet pills stuffed with desiccated road kill. And I wanted it to be fun to read: most books on wellness topics are duller than fifth grade geography.

Let's reprise. We started in a place to which I've never seen other diet 'experts' go: I urged you not to start dieting. Instead, I suggested that you stop dieting and concentrate on regaining control of your body, by beginning a modest exercise program and by reducing the sugar in your diet. Perhaps the most important lesson in the entire book is this: you must learn how to maintain your weight before you try to lose anything. Losing weight is hard, but keeping those pounds off is brutal. If you take your time, that brutal job becomes second nature, and managing your weight loss becomes just another of Life's tasks. It's like cleaning up after your dog – while you're doing it, you think of something else. But you do it every day.

While you were learning maintenance, I suggested that you (1) choose your diet intelligently, and (2) plan how you would live your life once you decided to stop losing more weight. The time to plan for your future body is now – today! – not some fuzzy point in the future when a thinner you struggles against a tide of nightmares trying to suck you back into the netherworld of out-of-control eating.

Survival Skills

Just after the introduction, I listed ten of the survival skills we all need in a world in which food is thrust at us from every direction. I also listed the outline of The 16-Word Diet program:

1. <u>STOP GAINING WEIGHT</u>. Don't go on a diet immediately. instead, learn how to stop gaining weight. If you don't, then what will you do when you stop dieting?

2. <u>START TO EXERCISE.</u> If you do not exercise, now is the time to start. People who do not exercise look unhealthy and undesirable. What good is a diet if you end up thinner but remain unhealthy and undesirable? Why exercise first and diet second? Because you can start exercising

right now. You'll feel better almost immediately, and it will become an important part of learning how to not gain weight.

3. <u>SET REASONABLE GOALS</u>. Most people have completely unreasonable expectations about how much they should lose and how quickly they should lose it. If you want to maintain a weight loss, you need reasonable goals for both diet and exercise. Start by <u>learning your WeightZone,</u> and retest yourself every few months (regular exercise changes your Zone).

4. <u>SELECT THE DIET THAT IS BEST FOR YOU</u>. I recommend a protein-centered diet with little sugar and limited grains, but some people prefer a low-fat diet. Your body, your decision.

5. <u>LEARN THE 16-WORDS</u>. Start with the basic rules, then learn how to apply them to your life.

a. Eat reasonable portions of fresh, healthy foods.
b. Avoid processed foods and sugars.
c. Get regular, vigorous exercise.

6. <u>START TO DIET (AT LAST!)</u> I understand that this list sounds crazy – you want to start dieting this minute and lose all of your weight by Thursday. However, a diet is like a marathon run. If you do not train for it, you will fail. The first five steps were training; now you can start The 16-Word Diet.

7. <u>LEARN THE ART OF DIETING</u>. Yes, dieting is an art, difficult to master. The basics are easy: eat these foods, not those. But how do you handle stress? How do you regain control after you have overeaten for a few days or weeks?

8. <u>DON'T LOOK FOR MAGIC IN A BOTTLE</u>. Nothing sold over-the-counter works. It doesn't matter if it's diet supplements, diet pills, diet drinks, diet patches, diet extracts, or a book promising magic food combinations, they are 100% fake. However, there's a steady stream of liars promising that their new product works miracles.

9. <u>TRUST SCIENCE, NOT MYTHOLOGY</u>. This is essentially a generalization of the point above. The difference between science and mythology is that science keeps changing. New discoveries are often made which refine or even overturn long-held beliefs, and science absorbs the new discoveries, which makes it stronger. Mythologies, as alive and intelligent as a float in a Macy's Thanksgiving Day Parade, never change.

10. <u>LEARN TO FORGIVE YOURSELF WHEN YOU OVEREAT</u>. Of all the steps above, this is the hardest. I cannot write about it; I cannot teach it. However, this book can help you gain the wisdom to teach it to yourself.

Ten basic survival skills for dieters and just four are concerned with the specific foods you eat. The 16 Words – the heart of this program! – are fifth on the list, not first. Why? Because food is at best forty percent of the problem that we dieters face every day. 60% is about coping with life every day, even every hour. That's why I wrote this book. I hope you learned from it, and enjoyed it.

One last note. If you haven't already done so, go to www.weightzonefactor.com, fill out the questionnaire, and leave your email address for me. That will register you to get Jay's Blog every week, and make it easy to contact me if you have questions. Good luck!

ঙঙঙঙঙ

Appendix

Why WeightZone Gives Better Advice than the BMI

The Body Mass Index is one of the most widely used measurements in medicine. It is also the most inaccurate.

Think about that. Scientists can determine your ideal temperature and heart rate with breath-taking precision, but they have no clue about how much you should weigh. The devices that measure body fat percentage offer a slight help to the profoundly clueless, but that is about as good as it gets.

Here's the reality. You want to know two things about your weight: how much you should weigh to improve your chances of living as long as possible, and how much you should weigh to look your best. No, they are not the same thing, and that is where matters get complicated. As I explained elsewhere in this book: people who are a little 'overweight' by societal standards live longer than thinner people. That's one reason that WeightZone gives you a range of weight, not just a magic number. You look better at the low end, but live longer at the upper end. Your call.

WeightZone gives custom results to every user; the BMI assumes that everyone who is the same height should be at the same weight. Men, women, old, young, if their height is the same, the BMI says their weight should be the same. As a result, broad people, muscular people, tall people, almost everyone who is not small-framed and shorter than average is branded as being overweight by the *BMI – even if they are at a healthy weight!*

Think about this: I am 5′ 10″ (177.8 cm) with an unusually broad, muscular frame. My mother was a slender, sedentary 5′ 10″ woman. According to the Body Mass Index, since we were the same height, we should both have weighed the same amount: 153 (69.4 kg). And so should everyone else in the world who is 5′ 10″. In the real world, at 153 Mom would have been overweight and I would be dangerously underweight.

The Body Mass Index couldn't be worse if it had been invented by Congress.

The BMI is not supported by medical research. Adolphe Quetelet, a

Belgian mathematician, created the formula in 1832. In 1832, when leeches were used to cure people and surgeons didn't know that they had to wash their hands before surgery. Quetelet designed the BMI as a way to describe large populations and said repeatedly that his formula did not apply to individuals, but this didn't stop it from being used – or misused – in just that way. Almost 200 years later, doctors misuse the BMI with patients, trainers misuse it with clients, and worse, it is misused by those annoying weight charts that you see in many doctor's offices: those charts are based on the BMI and they give unhealthy advice.

The Insurance Industry Strikes Again

Decades ago, the BMI's tendency to tell many healthy people that they were overweight created a golden opportunity for the life insurance industry. Actuarial Trolls were dispatched to create a <u>weight chart</u> – a BMI-based chart that would make normal people look overweight when they applied for life insurance. Why? So that they could be charged higher premiums. The Actuarial Trolls had no interest in giving helpful advice to overweight people; they simply wanted to raise profits. Their system was brilliant:

1. Overweight people were claimed to be higher life insurance risks, despite the inconvenient fact that they lived longer than their thinner peers.

2. The Trolls built a weight chart with ludicrously small allowances for sex and frame size.

3. Because of the inaccurate chart, more than half of the people who applied for life insurance were tossed into the 'obese' category.

4. Rates went up.

That corrupt weight chart, over sixty years old and never updated, is still found in doctors' offices all around the country. It is a disgrace: doctors should know better. The Body Mass Index and weight charts have no place in modern medicine. If your doctor uses them and if you are anything but a small person who is not very muscular, run screaming from his office and find someone who does not use medical techniques from 1832.

WeightZone Gives Better Advice

We all need better advice. That is why I invented The WeightZone. I'm a mathematician; I designed WeightZone to be more accurate and more useful than the BMI. WeightZone is powered by an algorithm that analyzes 25 different factors: body statistics, health history, and exercise history. It tells me that my ideal WeightZone is between 204 and 214. If I weigh more than 214, my chances for heart disease, stroke, and diabetes may go up. If I weigh much less than 204, I might become underweight. I'd operate below my peak and be less able to fight off wasting diseases such as cancer. Of course, if I reached my BMI – suggested weight of 153, I would be hospitalized.

WeightZone Gives Better Advice

We all need better advice. That is why, several years ago, I invented The WeightZone. I'm a mathematician; I designed WeightZone to be more accurate and more useful than the BMI. WeightZone is powered by an algorithm that analyzes 25 different factors: body statistics, health history, and exercise history. It tells me that my ideal WeightZone is between 204 and 214. If I weigh more than 214, my chances for heart disease, stroke, and diabetes may go up. If I weigh much less than 204, I might become underweight. I'd operate below my peak and be less able to fight off wasting diseases such as cancer. Of course, if I reached my BMI – suggested weight of 153, I would be hospitalized.

I exercise regularly. More exercise won't change my Zone, but if I ever stopped I'd need to lose 19 more pounds! How do I know? I used the WeightZone Calculator. It's a great tool. Scroll to the bottom of your Results Page and you'll see a button. (If you can't get to your Results Page, go back to **WeightZone** and retake your test.)

The BMI Formula

For those of you who still remember your high school math, here are the formulas – unchanged since Adolphe Quetelet created them in 1832:

$$BMI = (Weight \times 703) / Height^2$$
$$Weight = (BMI \times Height^2) / 703$$

Weight is in pounds; height is in inches. If you prefer metrics, simply remove the factor 703. Weight is in kg; height is in cm.

If you think that these formulas are not relevant to your body, you are not alone. They should have stayed in 1832.

Made in the USA
San Bernardino, CA
14 February 2018